THE OIL-CHANGE DIET

IMPROVE YOUR HEALTH AND LOSE WEIGHT BY CHANGING THE OIL YOU EAT

Print Edition

Available at Lulu.com

ISBN 978-1-312-36455-4

Table of Contents

Introduction to the Oil-Change Diet

My Story

For almost forty years, I have suffered from arthritis pain and taken non-steroidal anti-inflammatory drugs (NSAIDs). I also come from a family that lost many men to heart attacks in their fifties, so I have a personal interest in both arthritis and heart health. Additionally, because my mother, my wife, and my mother-in-law were diagnosed with diabetes, I'm concerned with that disease, as well.

My interest in diabetes led me to discovering this diet. During a casual conversation at a hunting-retriever test, an M.D. recommended the book *Protein Power* by Michael R. Eades, M.D., and Mary Ann Eades, M.D. My wife got the book and, by following its recommendations, she has done a great job of controlling her diabetes through her diet. She rarely has blood-sugar test results outside normal limits.

Protein Power has a chapter on lipids that my wife asked me to read and explain to her. This is how I began to learn about and develop an interest in understanding the effects of lipids in my own diet. Lipids are fat-like substances that the body uses to store energy and to make cells, hormones, and vitamins. Fatty acids are a basic type of lipid. Some fatty acids can be harmful in excess, such as LDL cholesterol and triglycerides. Others, such as essential fatty acids (EFAs), can be beneficial to health. In this book, we'll be talking primarily about two highly unsaturated fatty acids (HUFAs): omega-3 and omega-6. These EFAs have been getting a lot of attention regarding their roles as healthy fats in our diet. However, simply consuming more omega-3 EFAs is not the answer. What I have found through my research and through following this diet is that it is critical to consume the correct ratio of omega-3 to omega-6. That is the entire objective of the Oil-Change Diet.

I eventually found a National Institutes of Health (NIH) website and a downloadable program called KIM-2 (Keep It Managed-2). A graph illustrating the relationship between the lipids in our diet and heart attacks really grabbed my attention. I'll discuss the graph in more detail later, but the important thing to know now is that people from cultures that traditionally eat a healthy ratio of highly unsaturated fatty acids have a greatly reduced risk of heart attack.

After downloading and using the KIM-2 program and doing some additional research, I became convinced that changing the ratio of HUFAs in my diet could help me with my arthritis and blood pressure. Doing so was far more effective than I ever expected. I have been able to eliminate all of my medications: five different prescription drugs, a total of nine pills a day. An unexpected but desirable side effect of this diet was significant weight loss—I lost 15 pounds in just three weeks. I believe that most of this weight loss was a result of reduced inflammation and swelling. Since then I have lost an additional 45 pounds at a rate of about a pound a week (a healthier pace). This subsequent weight loss is the result of reduced appetite and decreased calorie intake resulting from the change in my diet.

The most important thing I learned in my research is the biochemistry and effects of the eicosanoids derived from the HUFA lipids in our bodies. These eicosanoids are super hormones, involved in all kinds of processes in our bodies. They affect almost everything! These super hormones—the prostaglandins, leukotrienes, thromboxanes, and lipoxins—are involved in regulating inflammation response, allergies, clotting, vasoconstriction, and bronchioconstriction, as well as many other important processes. Increasing your dietary intake of the right HUFAs (primarily omega-3 fatty acids) will increase the beneficial eicosanoids, and reducing your intake of the wrong HUFAs (omega-6 fatty acids) will reduce the eicosanoids that cause many of our health problems.

Due to my family history of heart attacks, I have tried to eat a healthy diet for over 30 years, avoiding eggs and red meat as major sources of cholesterol. When I first started getting cholesterol checked as part of my annual physical, it was obvious I had inherited some bad genes. My level of good cholesterol (HDL, or high-density lipoprotein) has always been lower than the recommended minimum of 40 mg/dl. However, even though I had been avoiding cholesterol and my level of bad cholesterol (LDL, or low-density lipoprotein cholesterol) was not very high, my LDL/HDL ratio was over 5, which is considered unhealthy. Improving my diet and taking statins reduced my total cholesterol to the range of 120–130 mg/dl, but my HDL remained below 40 mg/dl and the ratio stayed over 4. Even with a good diet and statins, my blood pressure became a problem a few years ago, so I started taking two different blood-pressure medications. By following the Oil Change Diet, I have been able to reduce my blood pressure enough to eliminate the need for any blood pressure medication. When I had a cholesterol test after eight months on this diet, my HDL was over 40 mg/dl for the first time ever (45 mg/dl) and my ratio was 3.9.

As I mentioned, I had taken NSAIDs since arthritis hit me in my late twenties. After almost 40 years, indomethacin, the NSAID that I had been taking for most of my adult life, just simply quit working. At times, the pain in my back was so severe, it would literally take my breath away; I couldn't breathe. My doctor changed my NSAID and added an additional pain reliever. After three weeks on the Oil Change Diet, I was able to eliminate the need for prescription NSAIDS. Now I take just an over-the-counter NSAID (like ibuprofen) when I do things that irritate my joints, like heavy lifting.

Any change in diet means learning to cook and eat differently. I started cooking when I was 13, after my mother went to Auburn for the summer, leaving my six younger brothers and me on our farm in Alabama. My dad was not a cook and was away working from early in the morning until about 5:00 p.m. I took over feeding the family. It didn't always go well. My brothers have never let me forget several of my cooking mistakes from that summer, but one in particular stands out.

I had helped my mom make gravy many times, stirring the flour as it browned in the frying pan after we fried something like chicken or pork chops. I knew she would just add some flour to the drippings in the pan and brown it a little before adding some milk or water to make the gravy. I did not know how much flour to add, so I asked my dad. He thought maybe a cup. So I browned about a cup of flour, but when I added the water, it turned into a huge lump of paste! I took about half of it out and added some more water. You could still slice the gravy.

Fortunately I kept improving, and I've helped my wife with cooking for most of our married years. As I retired before my wife did, she insisted that I take over all of the cooking duties. That was ten years ago.

With my large family, we have a lot of family gatherings. I do a lot of the cooking for them, but we have a lot of good cooks in the family who have taught me recipes and passed on tips. Seafood dishes like gumbos, shrimp Creole, and low-country boils are favorites in my family, and they are dishes that are high in good HUFAs. I don't claim to be a gourmet chef, but most of the people that have eaten my cooking seem to be willing to come back for more!

Cajun cooking and Mexican dishes are among my favorites, so obviously I like a lot of flavor. If you are not a fan of "heat" in your food, simply reduce or leave out the red pepper, jalapenos, and possibly some of the white pepper. Some of the recipes in this book are my own, some are favorites handed down from family and friends, and some are adapted from other sources.

Jump Start: The Oil-Change Diet in a Nutshell

Let me begin by saying that I am a retired research chemist in the field of marine science, not a physician. As I am a scientist, the science behind this diet is important to me. If you are interested in the science, it is here for you. I've made an effort to present the core of the information in a way that is easy to read and that non-scientists can understand, but this quick introductory section gives you the basics.

Again, I am not a medical doctor, so check with your doctor before making major changes to your diet or stopping any prescription medications. Consider the advice in this book, and then discuss your diet with your doctor. It may turn out that changing your oil will change your life!

This diet has one simple objective—decrease the ratio of omega-6 to omega-3 lipids in our bodies. (Lipids are a kind of fat.) In other words, you want to have more omega-3 and less omega-6. If you can get your ratio down to less than 50 percent, you will see significant health benefits, for example, your risk of heart attack will be cut by approximately 75 percent. The easy way to get to a healthy ratio is to eliminate all sources of vegetable oils, all nuts, and all grains. Read the ingredients list for all packaged foods; if there is any vegetable oil (like soybean oil, corn oil, even canola oil or olive oil), avoid it.

Fortunately, there are a few exceptions. You can use coconut oil and real butter for cooking, but if you want to lose weight, keep the quantity of fats down. A few nuts have levels of omega-6 lower than 70 percent, such as coconuts, macadamia nuts, and chestnuts. You can eat rice, bleached flour, and pasta because they have very little oil; however, eat them in moderation, since they increase insulin production, which in turn can increase the formation of harmful omega-6 lipids. Flax seed and chia seeds are beneficial. Don't worry about the omega-6 in veggies—most of them do not have very much omega-6 or omega-3 lipids in the first place, and they are loaded with many nutrients we need. Eat more fish and seafood, increase the protein in your diet, and reduce the fats and carbohydrates to lose weight. So that's it, simple and sweet! You can even have a few sweets; just avoid desserts that have vegetable oils, and don't overindulge.

You do not need to limit your diet choices to the recipes in this book; I encourage you to modify your own favorite recipes to avoid the vegetable oils and other foods that are high in omega-6. The food sections provide details about the levels of omega-6 in various food groups. Many recipes can be modified by replacing vegetable oils with coconut oil or butter. Add milled flax seed to your recipes to increase your intake of omega-3.

The recipe section has a variety of recipes for breakfast, lunch, and dinner, as well as some snack and dessert recipes. You will also find a month of daily menus to give you a guide to follow. I hope you will enjoy these recipes and find they help improve your health.

If you are curious about how and why these lipids make such a difference, I encourage you to read the rest of the introduction. These sections present the general science in a way that strives to be simple and clear. Then, if you want more detail, have a look at the appendices on lipids and eicosanoids near the end of this book. Those sections may be a little difficult if you are not scientifically inclined, but they still might be useful for helping you get to sleep! There is also a glossary and abbreviation section at the end that you can refer to if you need help with any of the terms or abbreviations.

***Why Follow This Diet?

Any diet worth following should improve your health. Better health was my goal, and I achieved it by changing the ratio of the lipids that are used to make eicosanoids, those cellular super-hormones, in every cell in my body—in other words, changing my oil from omega-6 to omega-3. These lipids (highly unsaturated fatty acid lipids, or HUFAs) are stored inside our cells as part of the cell membrane and are used to make the eicosanoid super hormones that control inflammation, clotting, allergies, and many other important functions. The ratio of omega-6 to omega-3 lipids in our cell membranes is dependent on the ratio of omega-6 and omega-3 lipids we eat. The good eicosanoids are derived from the omega-3 HUFAs. An excess of eicosanoids derived from omega-6 HUFAs will cause inflammation, which can be harmful to our health.

The information in this book and the KIM-2 program can be used with a variety of different dietary needs and preferences. Whether you are vegetarian, diabetic, or have other special needs, the sections on basic food information will be helpful to you. Weight loss alone will improve your health if you are overweight. Losing weight was not the original reason I started this eating plan, but that was one of the benefits. It is relatively high in protein, which tends to satisfy you longer and helps reduce hunger. In my case, the weight loss resulted mainly from my reduced appetite, but cutting out oils and nuts also reduced the calorie density of the food I ate. To lose weight on any diet, you must consume fewer calories than you burn. Your activity level determines how much you can consume each day. My activity level is fairly light, but I have been losing about a pound per week while eating approximately 1,500 calories per day. It is best to consume your calories in small amounts throughout the day rather than in one or two large meals. Don't eat until you are full; eat only what it takes to satisfy your hunger.

The real health benefits of this diet come from what is happening in your cells. By reducing the ratio of omega-6 to omega-3 lipids, we increase the probability of our cells making a beneficial hormone instead of one that promotes inflammation and damage. Each cell is surrounded by a double layer of lipid molecules. When a cell is stimulated to produce a hormone, it sends an enzyme (phospholipase, or PLA) to clip a HUFA molecule from that lipid bilayer. The PLA enzyme does not discriminate between omega-6 and omega-3 molecules. Therefore, the likelihood that a beneficial omega-3 molecule will get snipped and used in creating the hormone simply depends on the ratio of omega-6 and omega-3 HUFAs that make up your lipid bilayer. The typical American diet produces omega-6 to omega-3 ratios in excess of 4:1, or over 80 percent omega-6. We need to get that ratio down to 1:1 (50%) or slightly lower.

However, the relative ratio of omega-6 and omega-3 is not the only thing we should consider when we choose our foods. Consider all of the nutritional factors in the foods that you eat. Fruits and veggies contain vitamins, minerals, antioxidants, phytonutrients, polyphenols, fiber, and protein in addition to any omega-6 or omega-3 fats they may contain. All of these other components are important to our health. It is best to eat a variety of different foods, mainly fruits and vegetables, every day. Salads are a great way to increase the variety of foods you eat. You can make salads from a number of different greens, fruits, veggies, cheese, and meat, including fish and shellfish (which are good sources of omega-3 HUFAs). Smoothies are also a great way to consume a variety of fruits, and adding chia seeds or milled flax seed can enhance the omega-3 in them and in you.

The NIH website and the KIM-2 program use the term "percent long-6" to show the effects of various foods on the ratio of bad and good HUFAs in our bodies. "Percent long-6" refers to the percentage of omega-6 lipids in the 20- and 22-carbon HUFAs in our cells. (Fatty acids are primarily made up of a chain of carbon and hydrogen molecules, and each acid is defined by the number of carbon molecules and the number and location of double bonds between molecules.) The KIM-2 program calculates the percent long-6 based on the intake of long omega-6 and omega-3 HUFAs in the foods we eat and the conversion rates of short-chain (18-carbon) omega-3 and omega-6 essential fatty acids to long-chain (20- and 22-carbon) HUFAs in our bodies. The primary goal of this diet is to reduce the ratio of long omega-6 HUFAs in our cells to less than 50 percent. There are two ways to do that: increase the intake of omega-3, or reduce the intake of omega-6. We can increase our intake of omega-3 HUFAs by consuming more fish and shellfish or veggies high in omega-3. We can decrease our intake of omega-6 HUFAs by avoiding most common vegetable oils. These oils are high in short-chain omega-6 fatty acids, which are converted into long-chain omega-6 HUFAs. Oils such as soybean, corn, peanut, safflower—and even so-called healthy oils such as olive and canola—are high in short-chain omega-6 fatty acids. Just a tablespoon of some of these oils can contain as much as 10,000 mg of omega-6.

Fortunately, these short omega-6 fatty acids do not convert directly to long omega-6 HUFAs in a 1:1 ratio; rather, only a portion of the short omega-6 FAs become long omega-6 HUFAs. [1]

The long omega-6 HUFA that we are trying to reduce is arachidonic acid (AA). We consume this mainly in meats and dairy products, but it is also in fish and seafood in lower amounts. Most of the AA we consume is assimilated, and since it is already a HUFA, it does not need to be converted from an 18-carbon to a 20-carbon fatty acid. Meats contain long omega-3 HUFAs as well, some at near a 1:1 ratio, but often at less than 20 percent of the total, so we need to be careful in our selection of meats and reduce the portion size as much as possible. Meats from grass-fed animals are more likely to have an omega-6/omega-3 ratio near 1:1 than are grain-fed animals.

If you are vegan, you do not consume any long omega-6 or omega-3 HUFAs; your body must make them from the short omega-6 and omega-3 lipids that you consume. If you eat mainly fresh fruits, veggies, and legumes, and do not use vegetable oils or margarine for cooking, you will probably have a healthy omega-6/3 ratio. Vegetarians who consume eggs and dairy products get some long omega-6 and omega-3 lipids, but those lipids are close to balanced, especially if they come from grass-fed animals. However, whether you are a vegetarian or vegan, if you use vegetable oils and margarine in your cooking or eat a lot of nuts and fried snacks like potato chips, it is very likely you will have a high 6/3 ratio. It is important even for vegans and vegetarians to keep their omega-6/3 ratio in balance.

The first page of the KIM-2 program shows a graph [2] (shown below) of deaths related to heart disease and the association with the percent long omega-6 in their bodies. It was that graph that convinced me to try to reduce the omega-6 in my body. It shows that coronary heart disease causes 20 deaths per 100,000 in Greenland, where people have an average of 32 percent omega-6 HUFAs in their tissue. In Japan, the ratio of long omega-6 to long omega-3 HUFAs is less than 1:1 (50% omega-6), and fewer than 50 in 100,000 people die of heart disease. The US diet produces a ratio of more than 4:1 and has a heart-disease death rate of nearly 200 per 100,000. So, we want to keep our ratio close to 1:1, or lower if possible. The only medical problem that might be associated with getting the ratio of omega-6 to omega-3 too low (near or below 30%) is that it may increase the risk of bleeding and hemorrhagic strokes. [3]

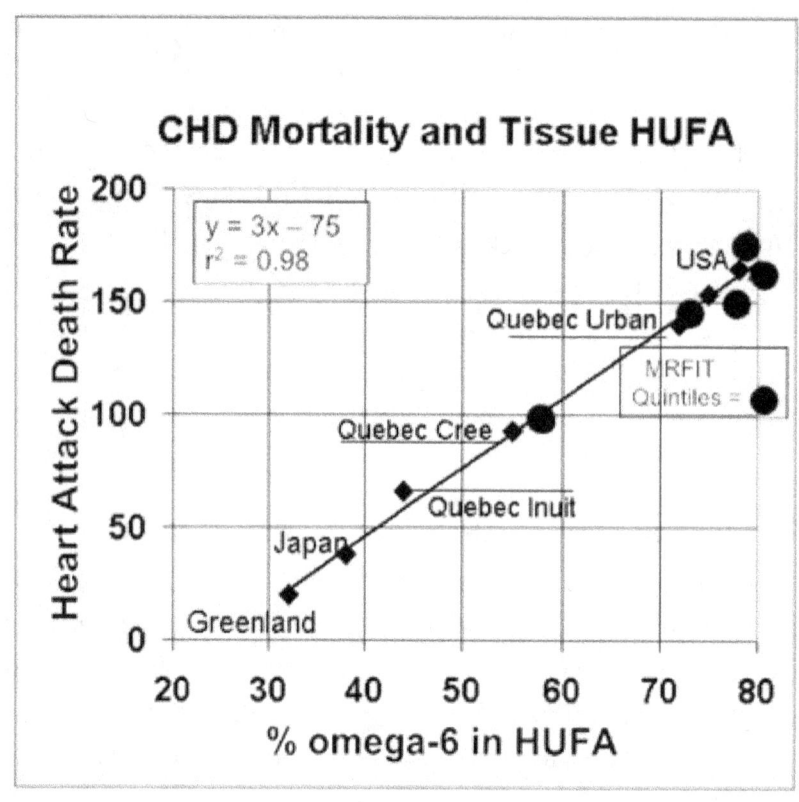

Omega-6 and Omega-3 PUFAs and HUFAs

The conversion of short-chain omega-6 and omega-3 poly-unsaturated fatty acids (PUFAs) into highly unsaturated fatty acids (HUFAs) is not straightforward. There is a complex formula that predicts the percent long omega-6 in our bodies. [4] The formula, revised in 2002 after adding information from hundreds of volunteers, uses eight constants derived from measurements of the percent long omega-6 and omega-3 HUFAs in the tissues of hundreds of individuals in the United States and Japan and the lipids in their diets. The KIM-2 program uses that formula to make predictions based on the foods we eat. I have used the KIM-2 program to calculate the percent long omega-6 we can expect in our tissues based on the foods in the recipes and menus in this book. The program also provides calorie and nutritional data that I include with each recipe. I have also provided omega-6 and lipid information on a series of food groups like meat, fish, fruits and veggies. Note that the percent of omega-6 in individual foods is not as important as the overall daily average of the percent long omega-6 HUFA produced by our diet. The key is the combination of the percent omega-6 and the overall calories in our food. For example, a red ripe tomato will produce 75 percent long omega-6, but if that tomato is just part of a day's diet that also included a small portion of salmon, the overall percent long omega-6 produced by your body that day will probably be below 50 percent.

I later found a more recent paper that provides a balance value for foods that takes into account their contribution to our daily calorie intake. [5] This balance value is much easier to understand and use. The balance score is based on a formula that takes into account the essential fatty acid content and nutritional content or calories in a food. It then generates a positive or negative integer. The more positive a balance score is, the better it is for lowering your omega-6/3 ratio; the more negative it is, the worse it is. Balance scores that are positive are considered good; those above 10 are considered very good. In the other direction, scores between 0 and –2 are considered acceptable; scores between –2 and –8 are poor; scores of –9 and higher are bad to awful. The list of balance scores and the app are available at http://fastlearner.org/. The KIM-2 program can be downloaded from http://efaeducation.org/sig/kim.html. [6]

In the food sections that follow, I provide lists of foods with the percent long omega-6 that they produce and their balance scores derived from the KIM-2 program and the balance score app. I encourage you to download and use the KIM-2 program and/or the balance score app so that you can make better choices when modifying your own recipes and improve your overall daily average intake of omega-3 foods. You can enter your own recipes into the KIM-2 program, and it will calculate the predicted omega-6 it will produces as well as calorie and overall nutritional data. You can see which ingredients are the sources of omega-6 and test alternate ingredients to learn how to modify the recipes to make them healthier.

Controlling Your Ratio of Omega-6 to Omega-3

This book provides recipes and menus that help you choose foods based on the level of long omega-6 HUFA they will produce in your body. Recipes and foods that lead to lower levels of long omega-6 HUFAs will help reduce inflammation, blood pressure, and allergy response. However, increasing your consumption of good foods is not enough, you really need to reduce the consumption of foods that increase your percent long omega-6 HUFAs. The foods you need to avoid are those that we have always been told are bad, like potato chips and fried foods, but the list also includes many foods we have always been told were healthy, like almonds, avocados, and olive oil.

The problem is that the percent omega-6 in some of the "bad" foods we need to avoid is so high that even a small amount can significantly increase your overall percent long omega-6, especially if you are not consuming high levels of fish and seafood. Most of the fruits and vegetables that are good for us do not contain very high levels of either good or bad oils; therefore, it only takes a small amount of other foods that are high in omega-6 or omega-3 fats to significantly shift our balance.

We have always heard it is best to eat a diet high in green leafy veggies, and that is true. Green leafy veggies contain more omega-3 fats than omega-6 fats, but their overall fat level is very low.

A cup of lettuce has only 90 mg of fat, contains almost three times more omega-3 than omega-6 fats, and will produce only 30 percent long omega-6 in our bodies. Add just one teaspoon of "good" olive oil and the percent long omega-6 it will produce in our bodies jumps to 68 percent. That is because the teaspoon of olive oil contains 356 mg of omega-6 but only 27 mg of omega-3 fatty acids.

"Bad" foods like potato chips contain almost 5,000 mg of omega-6 fatty acids in just one ounce, a 7-oz bag contains over 30,000 mg! Even a supposedly healthy snack food like peanuts contains over 4,400 mg of omega-6 fatty acid in just one ounce. There is ten times more omega-6 in just one ounce of peanuts or potato chips than there is omega-3 in a 3-ounce serving of most fish. That amount of omega-6 is twice as high as the amount of omega-3 even in salmon or mackerel, the fish that contain the highest levels of omega-3. Truly healthy snacks are plain fruits, maybe with a little cheese. One medium apple with an ounce of brie has just 265 mg of omega-6, and also has 114 mg of omega-3 fatty acids, producing only 55 percent long omega-6 in our bodies.

The food lists, recipes, and meal plans provided in this book will help you achieve the ratio of omega-6 and omega-3 HUFAs that you want to have in your body. A 50/50 ratio would be close to the diet of the Japanese people. In Japan, fewer than 50 deaths per 100,000 per year are due to heart disease, about one quarter the rate in the US. In addition, a 50/50 ratio will significantly improve our health in many other areas and, according to one study, would reduce our society's health-related medical costs by more than 50 percent.

It is difficult to overstate the implications of a healthy ratio. Inflammation and the damage it causes to cells have been linked to many of our most serious medical problems: heart disease, diabetes, cancer, Alzheimer's, arthritis, multiple sclerosis, irritable bowel syndrome, and many others. Without having done this research into the role of lipids in my wife's diabetes, I would have not believed that a diet could have had that much influence on my arthritis and blood pressure, and I would not have had the determination to make a commitment to changing my diet for long enough to see the effects myself. It took about three weeks of total avoidance of nuts, oils, and grains, and increasing my intake of fish and seafood, to be able to change my oil ratio and feel significantly better.

***

Oil Ratios in the Food Groups

Good Oils

There are only a few plant-based oils that contain significantly more omega-3 than omega-6 fatty acids: perilla oil (1,680 mg omega-6 and 8,960 mg omega-3 per tablespoon) and flaxseed oil (2,240 mg omega-6 and 7,980 mg omega-3 per tablespoon). These oils are not suitable for cooking, but can be used cold or taken in capsule form as dietary supplements. There are some other plant-based oils that contain relatively low levels of omega-6 fatty acids compared to most vegetable oils. Sunflower oil comes in two forms, high oleic oil (>70% oleic) or high linoleic (>70% linoleic). A tablespoon of the high oleic sunflower oil has only 505 mg of omega-6 fatty acid (plus 27 mg of omega-3), compared to 8,935 mg of omega-6 fatty acid in a tablespoon of high linoleic sunflower oil.

Coconut oil, palm kernel oil, and babassu oil are all relatively low in omega-6, with less than 250 mg of omega-6 fatty acids per tablespoon. Clarified or anhydrous butter is actually a lot better than most of our common cooking oils, with only 288 mg of omega-6 (plus 185 mg of omega-3) per tablespoon. However, while butter and these three oils are relatively low in omega-6 FA, they are high in saturated fats. Coconut oil is a medium-length saturated fat that does not contribute to LDL, and there is some evidence it can help increase HDL.

There is also a form of omega-6 oil (gamma linolenic acid or GLA) that can be converted to DGLA (di-homo-gamma-linolenic acid), which is a long omega-6 HUFA that is beneficial and anti-inflammatory. GLA occurs naturally in evening primrose, safflower, and borage oil, making up about 20 percent of the total fatty acids in these oils.

Fish oils are beneficial oils that contain both EPA and DHA, the beneficial omega-3 oils that we need to increase in our bodies. Whereas the natural form of fish oil is a triglyceride, most extracted fish oils are sold in an ester form that may not have the same effects. However, there are some forms of fish oil that are restored to the triglyceride form before being sold.

Bad Oils

Essentially all of the common cooking oils are made of predominantly omega-6 fatty acids, and they are produce very high levels of omega-6 HUFAs in our bodies. Common cooking oils like soybean, corn, and peanut oil are extremely high in omega-6 with very low levels of omega-3. Soybean oil has 6,936 mg of omega-6 per tablespoon; corn oil has 7,888 mg. Even so-called good oils, such as canola (2,842 mg omega-6, 1,302 mg omega-3 per tbs) and olive oil (1,067 mg omega-6, 81 mg omega-3 per tbs) have high ratios of omega-6 compared to omega-3.

Some nut oils, like walnut oil, do have a significant percentage of omega-3, but they still have much more omega-6 (7,194 mg omega-6, 1,414 mg omega-3 per tbs). Peanut oil has 4,320 mg of omega-6 per tbs, but no omega-3 at all. Similarly, both high linoleic and high oleic safflower oils are high in omega-6 while lacking any omega-3 (high linoleic: 10,149 mg omega-6 per tbs; high oleic: 1,952 mg of omega-6 per tbs). Sesame oil has 5,617 mg omega-6 and 41 mg omega-3 per tbs. Grapeseed oil has 9,466 mg of omega-6 but only 14 mg of omega-3 per tbs.

Margarine, even if it is made with canola oil and does not contain trans-fats, still contains high levels of omega-6. It is better to use real butter or even lard. Remember, though, that these are high in saturated fats and contain cholesterol that may be detrimental to heart health. I have been using a minimal amount of butter or coconut oil to replace oils in my cooking.

Fruits

Almost all fruits and veggies are relatively low in total omega-6 and omega-3 oils; however, avocados are high in omega-6 and low in omega-3, containing over 3,000 mg of omega-6 per fruit. Note that there is a difference between California and Florida avocados. California avocados are lower in omega-6 than Florida avocados, which contain over 4,000 mg of omega-6 and about 340 calories per fruit. However, California avocados contain a small amount of long omega-6 HUFAs and actually produce a slightly higher percent long omega-6 HUFAs in our bodies (79% compared to 75% for Florida avocados).

Even so, avocados provide many health benefits as they contain high levels of folate, potassium, carotenoids (like beta carotene, lutein, and zeaxanthin) and anti-inflammatory phytosterols. In addition, most of the oil in avocados is oleic acid, a mono-unsaturated fatty acid which cannot be converted to a long omega-3 or omega-6 HUFA and has been shown to reduce the conversion of short omega-6 into long omega-6 HUFAs. However, it is still probably best to keep the serving size small and not to eat them too frequently.

Below is a list of fruits and their fatty acid content, followed by a list with the percent long omega-6 they will produce in our bodies and their balance scores. Keep in mind that with the low amount of fatty acids in most fruit, balancing them with a small amount of foods high in omega-3 will keep our overall percent long omega-6 low.

Fruit	Omega-6 FA (mg)	Omega-3 FA (mg)	% Omega-6	Balance Score
Apple	120	25	61	–1
Avocado, Haas, 1 c	4,418	265	79	–9
Banana, 1 medium	66	39	44	0
Blueberries, 1 c	144	97	50	0
Cantaloupe, 1 c	73	98	39	0
Cherries, 1 c (with pits)	172	166	46	0
Grapes, 1 c	208	62	60	0
Kiwi, 1 c	365	62	67	–3
Mango	29	77	20	1
Melon, Casaba, 1c	29	37	35	0
Melon, Honeydew, 1 c	29	37	35	0
Nectarine	306	7	74	–2
Papaya, 1 c	8	35	15	1
Peach	43	1	62	–2
Pineapple, 1 c	130	96	49	0
Plum	88	0	72	–1
Strawberries, 1 c	156	112	52	0
Watermelon, 1 c	222	0	75	–2

Vegetables

The best veggies in terms of the percent long omega-6 they produce are the green leafy veggies that we have always heard are good for us. All veggies are relatively low in both omega-6 and omega-3, with the exception of green soybeans (edamame). Veggies are a great source of vitamins, minerals, and fiber, so even though some of these veggies individually may produce a relatively high percent long omega-6, consuming a variety of veggies is still a healthy choice since their total omega-6 is low. It is important to understand that point. Tomatoes, with 234 mg of short omega-6 per cup and producing 75 percent long omega-6 by itself, but consuming them as part of a dish like Shrimp Creole will result in just 36 percent long omega-6. This is because the dozen shrimp contain a total of 442 mg of long omega-3 HUFAs and only 73 mg of long omega-6 HUFA. Only a portion of the 234 mg of short omega-6 in the tomatoes will be converted to long omega-6, but most of the long omega HUFAs in the shrimp will be assimilated directly into our cells. (Technically, tomatoes are fruits, but since most of us think of them as vegetables, I've included them in this section.)

Here is a list of some common vegetables with their omega-6 and omega-3 content, followed by the percent omega-6 they produce in our bodies and their balance scores. Notice that the balance scores do not always increase with increasing percent omega-6 because the balance score takes into account the contribution to our total calorie intake.

Vegetable	Omega-6 FA (mg)	Omega-3 FA (mg)	% Omega-6	Balance Score
Asparagus, raw, 1 c	111	7	72	−2
Broccoli, raw, 1 c	33	114	24	3
Cabbage, raw, 1 c	36	48	46	0
Carrots, cooked, 1 c	119	17	64	−2
Cauliflower, cooked, 1 c	62	207	25	3
Celery, raw, 1 c	83	0	75	−5
Collards, cooked, 1 c	133	177	50	0
Corn, yellow, 1 ear, raw	488	14	75	−6
Cucumber, raw, 1 c	23	31	39	0
Edamame, cooked, 1 c	4,783	637	73	−12
Eggplant, cooked, 1 c	77	15	65	−2
Green Beans, raw, 1 c	25	40	34	2
Kale, raw, 1 c	92	121	46	0
Lettuce, Iceberg, 1 c	16	39	30	2
Onion, raw, 1 c	94	5	66	0
Peas, edible pod, raw, 1 c	47	8	63	−2
Pepper, bell, raw, 1 c	139	13	70	−2
Potato, baked	50	16	40	0
Spinach, raw, 1 c	7	35	17	3
Squash, yellow, cooked, 1 c	88	148	37	2
Tomato, raw 1 c	234	9	75	−4
Turnips, cooked, 1 c	31	88	26	2
Yam, raw, 1 c	96	18	49	0
Zucchini, raw, 1 c	27	46	36	2

Legumes

Peas and beans are high in protein and fiber and should be considered part of a healthy diet. However, there are a few legumes like soybeans, chickpeas, pigeon peas and fava beans that we should limit in our diet since they are relatively high in omega-6. Here is a list of legumes with the omega-6 and omega-3 content followed by the predicted percent omega-6 that they will produce in our bodies and the balance scores.

Legume	Omega-6 FA (mg)	Omega-3 FA (mg)	% Omega-6	Balance Score
Black beans	644	539	44	0
Chickpeas	5,186	202	75	−4
Cranberry beans	560	468	43	0
Fava beans	872	69	66	−1
Kidney beans	178	280	27	0
Lima beans, large	383	169	47	0
Mung beans	739	56	61	−1
Navy beans	626	524	43	0
Peas, split	810	165	59	−1
Peas, green, raw	220	51	62	−1
Peas, pigeon	1,595	72	69	−2
Pinto beans	328	457	33	0
Soybeans	18,461	2,474	73	−19

Nuts

Nuts are one of my favorite foods and something I always thought was healthy. Unfortunately, most nuts are high in omega-6. While nuts may be high in protein and nutrients, their high omega-6 content has led me to largely eliminate them from my diet. There are a few that are not too bad, like coconuts, macadamia nuts, and chestnuts, so, if you do want to consume some nuts, you should choose those that have a low balance score and keep the quantity down.

Here is a list of various nuts with the omega-6 and omega-3 content followed by the predicted percent long omega-6 that they will produce in our bodies and their balance score.

Nut	Omega-6 FA (mg)	Omega-3 FA (mg)	% Omega-6	Balance Score
Almonds	17,344	0	79	−21
Cashews, dry-roasted	10,494	221	77	−13
Chestnuts, European	1,110	133	69	−3
Coconut meat	293	0	63	−1
Hazelnuts	9,008	100	78	−13
Macadamia nuts	1,737	276	64	−2
Peanuts, oil-roasted	22,429	4	79	−21
Pecans, raw	24,807	1,134	77	−28
Walnuts, English	45,712	10,896	69	−44
Walnuts, black	41,340	2,508	77	−50

Fish and Seafood

Probably the easiest way to reduce our percent long omega-6 is to consume more fish and seafood. (Just make sure it is not fried!) All seafood contains EPA and DHA, the long omega-3 HUFAs that turn into beneficial eicosanoids. Some fish and seafood are higher than others in these beneficial HUFAs, like salmon and mackerel. Some fish, like bluefish and striped bass, contain almost no omega-6 and produce a very low percent long omega-6 in our bodies. However, in addition to omega-3 HUFAs, some seafood and fish contain significant amounts of omega-6 HUFAs, and some contain small amounts of short omega-6 and omega-3 fatty acids. The following list shows the amount of long omega-6 and long omega-3 HUFAs as well as the predicted percent long omega-6 HUFA they will produce.

Seafood	Omega–6 FA (mg)	Omega–3 FA (mg)	% Omega–6	Balance Score
Bass, freshwater	122	577	38	33
Bass, striped	0	641	0	55
Bluefish	0	708	1	48
Caviar, black or red, 1 oz	143	1,919	22	166
Catfish	127	394	47	–3
Clams	35	165	29	15
Cod, Atlantic	19	165	17	9
Fish sticks, frozen, 1 serv	10	125	55	–7
Flounder	32	208	23	26
Grouper	48	225	28	12
Halibut	118	388	43	15
Herring, kippered, 1 oz	23	621	12	70
Mackerel, Atlantic	156	2,134	21	33
Mullet, striped	82	360	36	14
Mussels	60	394	29	32
Oysters, eastern, 1 cup	198	1,543	30	43
Pollock	22	377	13	32
Salmon, Atlantic	227	1,465	35	73
Sardine, canned in oil, 1 oz	0	278	26	19
Scallop	20	183	16	no value given
Shrimp	74	447	30	4
Tuna, canned in water	29	237	18	46
Tuna, light, canned in oil	0	109	58	–9
Tuna, yellowfin	24	196	17	6

Meats

Meats do not contain appreciable amounts of omega-3 HUFAs, but they do contain arachidonic acid, the long omega-6 HUFA that is the precursor of the bad eicosanoids and both omega-6 and omega-3 fatty acids. Even lean meat will produce high percentages of long omega-6 in our bodies due to the fact that the cell membranes of animal tissue contain arachidonic acid. When we consume this acid, it is assimilated directly into our bodies.

Lean meats are lower in overall quantity of omega-6 as well as unsaturated fats and cholesterol. Animal fat is generally considered unhealthy. White-meat chicken is lower in omega-6 than dark meat, and both are lower when skinless. However, even white meat will produce 81 percent long omega-6 in our bodies. Roasted white-meat turkey with no skin is a little better, producing just 60 percent long omega-6. Lean meat portions of beef, such as eye of round, will produce about 70 percent long omega-6. Pork loin, even without fat, produces a 92 percent long omega-6; however, lean ham steak will produce only 70 percent omega-6.

Domestic, farmed meats often contain higher levels of omega-6 due to the grains that they are fed. Wild game, grass-fed beef, and free-range chickens contain comparatively lower amounts of these omega-6 fatty acids. For instance, a portion of roasted venison round will produce only 57 percent long omega-6. The bottom line is that consumption of meats should be minimized if you are trying to reduce the percent long omega-6 in your body. Keep portions small—3 to 4 oz— and avoid skin and fat. The list below shows the amount of these lipids and the predicted percent long omega-6 they will produce in our bodies. Note that the formula used for these predictions is obviously not perfect, since some of these predictions are over 100 percent. In these instances, just consider that as an indication that that food will significantly increase our overall omega-6 HUFAs in our bodies.

Meat	Omega–6 FA (mg)	Omega–3 FA (mg)	Omega–6 HUFA (mg)	% Omega–6	Balance Score
Beef, chuck, cooked	255	34	51	97	-2
Beef, skirt steak, broiled	417	51	43	88	-2
Beef, T-bone, broiled	490	241	20	63	-2
Chicken, dark meat, roasted	781	37	51	101	-6
Chicken, white meat, roasted	319	14	46	97	-4
Chicken, white meat, fried	6,091	338	132	93	-10
Duck, wild, raw	423	58	0	63	no value given
Pork, ham steak, cured	366	34	0	70	-3
Pork, loin, braised	884	34	34	91	-5
Pork, sausage patty, cooked	886	143	0	70	no value given
Turkey, white, roasted	263	5	79	99	-3
Venison, loin, broiled	50	23	14	53	-1

All entries are for 3 oz.

It is worth noting Omega-3 HUFA levels for some meats:

> Chicken, breast with skin, batter-fried: 75 mg omega-3 HUFA
> Chicken, skinless breast, roasted: 18 mg long omega-3 HUFA
> Chicken, dark meat from ½ chicken, roasted: 32 mg long omega-3 HUFA
> Turkey, skinless breast, roasted: 28 mg long omega-3 HUFA

Dairy and Egg Products

Most dairy fats are higher in short omega-6 fatty acids than short omega-3, but the percent long omega-6 they produce in our bodies is generally only slightly above 50 percent. Even real butter only produces about 53 percent long omega-6. Dairy fats do contain additional saturated fats and cholesterol that have been associated with coronary artery and heart disease, so it is best to keep dairy fat intake low. However, dairy products are a great source of calcium and protein. In addition, dairy products seem to have weight-reducing benefits. Fortunately, there are many fat-free dairy products. Fat-free cottage cheese and fruit is a tasty and healthy start to the day, as is low-fat yogurt with fruit. Skim milk and low-fat milk are also great low-omega-6 additions to a healthy meal, providing both calcium and protein.

Even eggs are available fat- and cholesterol-free. Omelets made from liquid egg-white products with vegetables such as mushrooms, green peppers, or spinach, are low in calories and high in protein.

There are a few cheeses that are slightly higher in omega-3 than omega-6, like Parmesan and Romano. They produce about 39 percent long omega-6 HUFAs. Cheese and fruit make an appetite-suppressing snack and can produce a percent long omega-6 of less than 50 percent, depending on the fruit.

Here is a list of dairy products and their omega-6 and omega-3 content followed by their predicted percent omega-6 they will produce and their balance scores.

Dairy Product	Omega-6 FA (mg)	Omega-3 FA (mg)	% Omega-6	Balance Score
Cheeses				
Blue, 1 oz	152	75	53	–1
Brie, 1 oz	145	89	51	–1
Cheddar, 1 oz	164	103	50	–1
Cottage cheese, nonfat, 4 oz	12	5	24	0
Cottage cheese, 2%, 4 oz	47	19	43	–1
Cream cheese, 1 oz	219	139	52	–1
Feta, 1 oz	92	75	46	0
Goat, soft, 1 oz	142	0	70	–2
Gouda, 1 oz	75	112	35	0
Parmesan, 1 oz	77	84	38	0
Romano, 1 oz	81	88	39	0
Mozzarella, part-skim, 1 oz	95	39	54	1
Ricotta, part-skim, 1 oz	54	20	56	–1
Swiss, 1 oz	176	100	52	–1
Other dairy				
Butter, 1 tbs	260	168	53	–3
Cream, half-and-half, 1 oz	79	50	52	–1
Egg, whole, I large	574	17	114	–17
Egg whites, 1 c	0	0	0	no value given
Yogurt, plain, nonfat, 8 oz	9	2	16	0

Grains and Cereals

Almost all grains in raw form contain significant amounts of short omega-6 fatty acids that turn into the long omega-6 HUFAs we need to reduce in our diets. Many of these grains are the source of the oils we are trying to avoid, like corn and soybean oil. Even wheat germ oil contains over 7,400 mg of omega-6 per tablespoon. In addition, when most of the cereals and grains are used to make bread, snacks, dry cereals, or pastries, we add additional oils. Snacks such as extruded corn-based chips are extremely bad, with over 4,000 mg of omega-6 per ounce. A 7-ounce bag has about 30,000 mg of omega-6. Even granola bars, depending on the type, can be loaded with over 3,000 mg of omega-6.

There are only two breakfast cereals that have balance scores in the good range: Uncle Sam Cereal and Nature's Path Optimum. There are a few more that fall into the acceptable range, including my favorite, grits. Pasta is probably one of the best forms of grain in most normal diets. Pasta is essentially 100 percent carbohydrates, with no added oils, and generally contains only a little over 300 mg of omega-6 per cup of cooked pasta. Vegetable-based pastas, such as spinach pasta, are even better. Enriched white flour is also pretty low in omega-6 since the wheat germ containing most of the omega-6 has been removed. So, breads like French breads that do not contain added oil are not bad. Whole-wheat breads contain the wheat germ, which does contain the natural oils from wheat. Typical commercial breads contain between 200 and 500 mg of omega-6 FA per serving. However, bread that contains added oil should be avoided.

One other way I often use flour is to make roux for gumbos and etouffeé. Since these dishes contain a lot of seafood, the balance ratio is good. I also provide several recipes for bread, tortillas, crackers, and biscuits with added flax that are higher in omega-3 than omega-6. White rice is also relatively low in total omega-6, with less than 100 mg per cup of cooked rice. However, grains are also high in carbohydrates, and the metabolism of carbohydrates requires insulin. The presence of insulin reduces the conversion of some of the shorter C-18 omega-3 oils into the beneficial omega-3 HUFAs. So, if you want to reduce the percent long omega-6 HUFAs in your body, it is best to keep your intake of grains and cereals as low as possible.

There are a few grains that contain more omega-3 oils than omega-6, such as flax seeds and chia seeds. I will discuss these super foods in the next section, but they are included here with a list of grains and cereals with their omega-6 and omega-3 content followed by the % omega-6 they produce in our bodies and their balance scores.

Cereal Product	Omega–6 FA (mg)	Omega–3 FA (mg)	% Omega–6	Balance Score
Blueberry muffin, 1 med	2,601	168	80	−18
Bread, white, 1 slice	425	50	71	−3
Bread, whole wheat, 1 slice	216	11	72	−2
Cheerios, 1 c dry	322	20	71	−4
Chia seeds, 1 oz	911	1,096	44	24
Corn Flakes, 1 c dry	109	3	63	0
Cornmeal, 1 c dry	1,939	60	74	−4
Crackers, snack, 3 crackers	1,064	79	75	−21
Cream of wheat, 1 c	1,282	154	66	−1
Flax seeds, 1 oz	1,036	4,349	22	32
Flour, white enriched, 1 c	489	28	62	−1
Flour, whole wheat, 1 c	886	42	70	−3
Graham cracker, 1 oz	1,010	73	74	−8
Granola, 1 c dry	1,827	102	72	−6
Grits, 1 c dry	764	16	65	−1
Macaroni, 1 c dry	621	59	65	−1
Oats, instant, 1 c dry	1,804	100	74	−7
Pie crust, frozen, 1/8	606	39	74	−7
Rice, white, 1 c dry	270	57	44	0
Rice, brown 1 c dry	1,850	81	71	−2
Sesame seeds, 1 tbs	1,924	34	78	−36
Spaghetti, 1 c, cooked	349	34	66	−1

Special Items

Flax and chia seeds are exceptions among the grains. They both contain more omega-3 than omega-6. Chia seeds have a unique ability to create a gel or pudding when mixed with water, hot or cold. Both are high in protein and fiber. The oils in both of these are easily oxidized, and care should be taken to avoid oxidation. That is, they should be kept fresh (don't store them for long periods) and stored in a cool, dark place.

Milled flax seed is a very powerful tool in this diet. It can be eaten raw and sprinkled on top of prepared foods, salads, and yogurt, or it can be added to foods before cooking. It does not alter the taste or texture of the foods significantly in either case, but it can significantly change the balance of the omega-3 and omega-6 fats in the food. Milled flax even comes in convenient travel packets that can be used to significantly reduce the percent omega-6 in foods when we are eating out at restaurants.

There is also a pasta called shirataki pasta that contains zero calories. It is made from the roots of the *Amorphophallus Konjak* plant, also called the konnayku imo. The root of the plant is similar to, but not related to, a yam and contains a non-digestible soluble fiber called glucomannan. The pasta contains no carbs and no fat. It is best used in soups and stir-fry dishes.

Seaweeds and algae are the source of omega-3 fatty acids and HUFAs in fish and seafood. Seaweeds do not contain much fat, but what little is there is the type that leads to lower omega-6 HUFAs in our bodies. One tablespoon of wakame seaweed (dried) contains 10 mg of long omega-3, Irish moss contains 5 mg of long omega-3, and laver contains 4 mg long omega-3— and each of these have less than 1 mg of long omega-6. Consider adding small amounts of re-hydrated seaweeds to your soups and salads.

***

Recipes

All the recipes in this book serve 1, unless otherwise stated.

Breakfast

Cottage Cheese with Mixed Berries

> 4 oz cottage cheese (nonfat)
>
> 2 oz blueberries
>
> 2 oz blackberries
>
> 2 oz strawberries
>
> 1 tbs milled flax seed
>
> Zero-calorie sweetener (optional)

Fresh berries are best in this, of course, but thawed frozen berries are a good alternative. Slice any large berries and mix them with the cottage cheese. Sprinkle with milled flax seed and zero-calorie sweetener if desired.

Calories per Serving	Calcium (mg)	Folate (mcg)	Zinc (mg)	Fiber (g)	Protein (g)	Predicted % Omega-6
166	63	49	1	5	21	29

Overall Fat (g)	Saturated Fat (g)	Cholesterol (mg)	Short Omega-6 (mg)	Short Omega-3 (mg)	Long Omega-6 (mg)	Long Omega-3 (mg)
2	0	8	314	803	0	0

Without the flax seed, the calories drop to 146, but the percent long omega-6 increases to 48%.

Egg-White Omelet

Whites from 4–6 large eggs or ½ c commercially prepared liquid egg whites

1 tbs onion, finely chopped

1 tbs green peppers, finely chopped

1 medium mushroom, chopped

1 oz cheddar cheese, shredded

1 tsp butter

If you are using fresh eggs, separate the yolks (you can save these to use in other recipes) and whip them briefly with a fork or spatula. Melt 1 tsp butter in a small nonstick pan over medium heat. Pour eggs into pan, add shredded cheese, and cook until the eggs are brown on bottom. In a separate pan, sauté the onions, peppers, and mushrooms in 1 tsp butter. Add sautéed veggies to eggs and fold over.

Calories per Serving	Calcium (mg)	Folate (mcg)	Zinc (mg)	Fiber (g)	Protein (g)	Predicted % Omega-6
204	216	15	1	1	21	51

Overall Fat (g)	Saturated Fat (g)	Cholesterol (mg)	Short Omega-6 (mg)	Short Omega-3 (mg)	Long Omega-6 (mg)	Long Omega-3 (mg)
12	7	35	248	134	0	0

Without cheese, this omelet is just 72 calories and produces 52% omega-6.

Blueberry Oatmeal with Flax Seed

¼ c oatmeal, regular or quick-cooking

¼ c blueberries, frozen

1 tsp butter

1 tbs milled flax seed

½ c water

Mix all ingredients and cook in microwave for 2 minutes.

Calories per Serving	Calcium (mg)	Folate (mcg)	Zinc (mg)	Fiber (g)	Protein (g)	Predicted % Omega-6
193	38	42	1	6	6	34

Overall Fat (g)	Saturated Fat (g)	Cholesterol (mg)	Short Omega-6 (mg)	Short Omega-3 (mg)	Long Omega-6 (mg)	Long Omega-3 (mg)
10	3	11	1,091	2,278	0	0

Without the flax seed, the oatmeal is 134 calories but will produce 68% omega-6.

Scrambled Egg Whites with Cheese

¼ c egg whites or liquid eggs

1 oz cheddar cheese

1 c skim milk

salt and pepper to taste

Scramble the eggs whites with the cheese and cook in a nonstick pan over medium heat to desired doneness. I like to brown the eggs and cheese slightly to add some flavor. Season with salt and pepper.

Calories per Serving	Calcium (mg)	Folate (mcg)	Zinc (mg)	Fiber (g)	Protein (g)	Predicted % Omega-6
230	509	19	2	0	22	46

Overall Fat (g)	Saturated Fat (g)	Cholesterol (mg)	Short Omega-6 (mg)	Short Omega-3 (mg)	Long Omega-6 (mg)	Long Omega-3 (mg)
10	6	35	176	108	0	0

With 8 oz orange juice:

Calories per Serving	Calcium (mg)	Folate (mcg)	Zinc (mg)	Fiber (g)	Protein (g)	Predicted % Omega-6
256	235	81	1	0	15	48

Overall Fat (g)	Saturated Fat (g)	Cholesterol (mg)	Short Omega-6 (mg)	Short Omega-3 (mg)	Long Omega-6 (mg)	Long Omega-3 (mg)
10	6	30	235	131	0	0

Flax Pancakes

¾ c self-rising flour

¼ c milled flax seed

¼ c egg whites or liquid eggs

2 tbs non-fat dry milk

½ c water

tsp sugar (optional)

Mix all ingredients together and add water to desired consistency. You may not need the whole amount. If you like, you can add the sugar to enhance browning. Spoon batter into a non-stick pan; turn when bubbles appear on top and pancake is brown on bottom. Makes 4–5 servings of 2 pancakes.

Calories per Serving	Calcium (mg)	Folate (mcg)	Zinc (mg)	Fiber (g)	Protein (g)	Predicted % Omega-6
154	71	75	1	3	7	24

Overall Fat (g)	Saturated Fat (g)	Cholesterol (mg)	Short Omega-6 (mg)	Short Omega-3 (mg)	Long Omega-6 (mg)	Long Omega-3 (mg)
4	0	1			0	0

I often have these pancakes with a couple spoonfuls of fruit salad instead of butter and syrup; however, for comparison here is the nutritional information for the pancakes with 2 tsp of real butter and 2 tbs of reduced calorie syrup:

Calories per Serving	Calcium (mg)	Folate (mcg)	Zinc (mg)	Fiber (g)	Protein (g)	Predicted % Omega-6
239	72	75	1	3	7	26

Overall Fat (g)	Saturated Fat (g)	Cholesterol (mg)	Short Omega-6 (mg)	Short Omega-3 (mg)	Long Omega-6 (mg)	Long Omega-3 (mg)
8	3	12	602	1,820	0	0

Traditional Pancake Breakfast

For further comparison, listed below is the omega-6, calorie, and nutritional information from KIM-2 for a traditional pancake breakfast with bacon and orange juice.

3 six-inch pancakes, plain

3 strips bacon, pan fried

2 tsp margarine (corn oil)

3 tbs maple syrup

8 oz orange juice

Calories per Serving	Calcium (mg)	Folate (mcg)	Zinc (mg)	Fiber (g)	Protein (g)	Predicted % Omega-6
936	577	165	5	0	22	80

Overall Fat (g)	Saturated Fat (g)	Cholesterol (mg)	Short Omega-6 (mg)	Short Omega-3 (mg)	Long Omega-6 (mg)	Long Omega-3 (mg)
36	9	152	11,214	1,374	66	12

Lunch

Tomato, Cucumber, and Onion Salad

½ c onion, thinly sliced

½ c sliced tomato

½ c sliced cucumber

1 oz feta cheese

¼ c vinegar

Mix the onion, tomato, cucumber, and feta, and pour vinegar over the salad. Add salt and pepper to taste.

Calories per Serving	Calcium (mg)	Folate (mcg)	Zinc (mg)	Fiber (g)	Protein (g)	Predicted % Omega-6
131	168	42	1	2	6	57

Overall Fat (g)	Saturated Fat (g)	Cholesterol (mg)	Short Omega-6 (mg)	Short Omega-3 (mg)	Long Omega-6 (mg)	Long Omega-3 (mg)
7	4	25	259	103	0	0

If you add just 1 tbs of olive oil, the percent long omega-6 predicted will jump to 70 percent and the calories to 250. If you want to increase the omega-3, you can add a small amount of milled flax seed or flaxseed oil.

Salad with Sardines

  1 c chopped lettuce

  ½ c chopped tomato

  1 tbs chopped onion

  ¼ c sliced cucumber

  ¼ c chopped green pepper

  1 oz feta cheese

  2 sardines

  zero-calorie salad dressing

Mix salad ingredients and top with sardines. Use a zero calorie salad dressing. I like Walden Farms brand Honey Mustard.

Calories per Serving	Calcium (mg)	Folate (mcg)	Zinc (mg)	Fiber (g)	Protein (g)	Predicted % Omega-6
257	375	81	2	3	18	37

Overall Fat (g)	Saturated Fat (g)	Cholesterol (mg)	Short Omega-6 (mg)	Short Omega-3 (mg)	Long Omega-6 (mg)	Long Omega-3 (mg)
16	7	72	371	359	259	1,272

It is surprising how well sardines go with salad. Serving them this way eliminates the need for snack crackers, which are high in omega-6 fats. Other seafood items, such as shrimp or smoked salmon, also go well with salad and can be used to increase the omega-3 content in your diet.

Salmon Patties

　　1 16-oz can pink salmon, drained

　　¼ c chopped onion

　　¼ c chopped celery

　　½ c egg whites or liquid eggs

　　½ c seasoned breadcrumbs

　　½ tsp salt

　　¼ tsp pepper

Mix all ingredients and form into patties. Brown in nonstick pan over medium-high heat (use cooking spray or a small amount of butter if necessary). Makes 8 patties; serves four.

Calories per Serving	Calcium (mg)	Folate (mcg)	Zinc (mg)	Fiber (g)	Protein (g)	Predicted % Omega-6
282	280	54	1	2	29	13

Overall Fat (g)	Saturated Fat (g)	Cholesterol (mg)	Short Omega-6 (mg)	Short Omega-3 (mg)	Long Omega-6 (mg)	Long Omega-3 (mg)
8	2	63	267	232	87	1,928

Fish Soup

 1 c fish stock

 3 oz cooked fish (broiled or boiled), flaked

 2 tbs chopped green onion

 2 tbs shredded cabbage

 1 tbs carrots, sliced in thin slivers

 1 tbs seaweed like kelp or wakame, soaked and rinsed

 1 tbs sliced celery

 ½ c arugula

 ¼ c shirataki noodles

Combine fish stock, fish, vegetables, and noodles in a small saucepan. Bring to a boil, then lower heat and simmer until veggies are tender. Recipe is for one serving; multiply ingredients by the number of servings needed. Serve hot.

Calories per Serving	Calcium (mg)	Folate (mcg)	Zinc (mg)	Fiber (g)	Protein (g)	Predicted % Omega-6
171	76	101	1	1	28	26

Overall Fat (g)	Saturated Fat (g)	Cholesterol (mg)	Short Omega-6 (mg)	Short Omega-3 (mg)	Long Omega-6 (mg)	Long Omega-3 (mg)
3	1	42	78	50	77	479

Squash Soup

1 c chopped yellow squash

1 tsp butter

Salt and pepper to taste

Place squash in a boiler and cover with water, add butter and cook until tender. Puree squash with retained water. Serve hot.

Calories per Serving	Calcium (mg)	Folate (mcg)	Zinc (mg)	Fiber (g)	Protein (g)	Predicted % Omega-6
72	50	36	1	3	2	43

Overall Fat (g)	Saturated Fat (g)	Cholesterol (mg)	Short Omega-6 (mg)	Short Omega-3 (mg)	Long Omega-6 (mg)	Long Omega-3 (mg)
5	3	11	180	207	0	0

This soup is deliciously buttery!

Salad with Chicken or Shrimp

    1 c shredded romaine lettuce

    ¼ c chopped tomato

    ¼ c chopped cucumbers

    2 oz feta cheese

    2 tbs chopped green pepper

    1 tbs chopped onion

    3 oz roasted skinless chicken breast, shredded, or 3 oz cooked shrimp

    2 tbs vinegar or zero-calorie salad dressing

Mix all ingredients, top with vinegar or salad dressing.

With chicken:

Calories per Serving	Calcium (mg)	Folate (mcg)	Zinc (mg)	Fiber (g)	Protein (g)	Predicted % Omega-6
263	318	112	2	2	24	63

Overall Fat (g)	Saturated Fat (g)	Cholesterol (mg)	Short Omega-6 (mg)	Short Omega-3 (mg)	Long Omega-6 (mg)	Long Omega-3 (mg)
14	9	90	632	223	37	28

You can add a small amount of milled flax seed to reduce to percent omega-6.

With shrimp:

Calories per Serving	Calcium (mg)	Folate (mcg)	Zinc (mg)	Fiber (g)	Protein (g)	Predicted % Omega-6
268	344	114	3	2	28	28

Overall Fat (g)	Saturated Fat (g)	Cholesterol (mg)	Short Omega-6 (mg)	Short Omega-3 (mg)	Long Omega-6 (mg)	Long Omega-3 (mg)
13	9	216	307	214	60	285

Spinach and Feta Tortilla Pizza

    1 flax tortilla (see Breads)

    1 tsp garlic butter

    ¼ c cooked spinach

    ¼ c feta cheese

Brush the tortilla with the garlic butter. Arrange the spinach and cheese on the tortilla and bake for 5 to 6 minutes until it starts to brown. Slice and serve.

Calories per Serving	Calcium (mg)	Folate (mcg)	Zinc (mg)	Fiber (g)	Protein (g)	Predicted % Omega-6
301	416	209	3	4	14	33

Overall Fat (g)	Saturated Fat (g)	Cholesterol (mg)	Short Omega-6 (mg)	Short Omega-3 (mg)	Long Omega-6 (mg)	Long Omega-3 (mg)
17	10	57	555	555	1,145	0

Arugula, Tomato, and Feta Salad

   ½ c arugula leaves

   5 cherry tomatoes

   1 oz feta cheese

   1 tbs balsamic vinegar

Place chopped arugula leaves on salad plate, top with cherry tomatoes and feta cheese, and sprinkle with balsamic vinegar.

Calories per Serving	Calcium (mg)	Folate (mcg)	Zinc (mg)	Fiber (g)	Protein (g)	Predicted % Omega-6
97	161	32	1	1	5	57

Overall Fat (g)	Saturated Fat (g)	Cholesterol (mg)	Short Omega-6 (mg)	Short Omega-3 (mg)	Long Omega-6 (mg)	Long Omega-3 (mg)
6	4	25	216	96	0	0

This salad has only 97 calories and generates 57 percent long omega-6. If you add a teaspoon of milled flax seed, the omega-6 drops to 33 percent.

Black Bean Burger

    1 16-oz can black beans

    ½ c onions

    ½ c chopped bell pepper

    ¼ c egg whites or liquid eggs

    ½ c breadcrumbs

    ¼ c milled flax seed

    1 tsp cumin

    1 tsp chili powder

    ½ tsp hot sauce

    ½ tsp salt

Drain and mash black beans into a paste. Mix in remaining ingredients. Divide into 4 equal parts and shape into patties. Brown patties on a baking sheet at 375° for about 10 minutes per side.

Calories per Serving	Calcium (mg)	Folate (mcg)	Zinc (mg)	Fiber (g)	Protein (g)	Predicted % Omega-6
248	102	179	2	12	14	33

Overall Fat (g)	Saturated Fat (g)	Cholesterol (mg)	Short Omega-6 (mg)	Short Omega-3 (mg)	Long Omega-6 (mg)	Long Omega-3 (mg)
5	1	0	874	1,873	0	0

These are great topped with low-fat or fat-free sour cream. Even better, whip up some Sour Cream and Cilantro Spread (see recipe in Sauces, Dressings, and Seasonings).

Shrimp Cocktail

    3 oz shrimp, cooked

    ¼ c catsup

    ¼ c lemon juice

    1 tbs ground horseradish

    Dash Worcestershire sauce

    Dash hot sauce

Mix the liquid ingredients and the horseradish, and transfer to a serving bowl. Arrange the shrimp around the bowl and serve.

Calories per Serving	Calcium (mg)	Folate (mcg)	Zinc (mg)	Fiber (g)	Protein (g)	Predicted % Omega-6
167	66	24	1	1	18	28

Overall Fat (g)	Saturated Fat (g)	Cholesterol (mg)	Short Omega-6 (mg)	Short Omega-3 (mg)	Long Omega-6 (mg)	Long Omega-3 (mg)
2	0	129	152	28	74	447

Duck Breast Sandwich

  1 duck breast fillet

  2 tbs flour

  2 tbs bread crumbs

  2 tbs Parmesan cheese

  1 tbs coconut oil

  ¼ cup egg whites

  4-inch piece of flax French bread

  lettuce leaves

  Swiss cheese

  mustard

  pickled jalapeno peppers (optional)

Mix breadcrumbs and Parmesan cheese. Pound duck breast fillet until it is about ¼ inch thick. Coat with flour, dip in egg whites, and then in the breadcrumb mixture. Over medium heat, brown fillet in a pan with a small amount of coconut oil until coating is golden brown, 1–2 minutes per side. Split the French bread and spread with mustard. Serve the fillet on the bread, topped with a slice of Swiss cheese and lettuce. Garnish with jalapeno pepper slices and serve.

Calories per Serving	Calcium (mg)	Folate (mcg)	Zinc (mg)	Fiber (g)	Protein (g)	Predicted % Omega-6
808	365	252	3	8	48	40

Overall Fat (g)	Saturated Fat (g)	Cholesterol (mg)	Short Omega-6 (mg)	Short Omega-3 (mg)	Long Omega-6 (mg)	Long Omega-3 (mg)
23	11	90	1,908	2,629	0	0

This is one of my favorite sandwiches. It has only 40% omega-6 due to the omega-3 in the French bread. You can substitute venison, veal, or even chicken in place of the duck.

Imitation Crab with Sour Cream Cilantro Sauce

    4 oz of Louis Kemp Crab Delights (imitation crab made with Alaskan pollock)

    1 tbs of Sour Cream Cilantro Sauce (see Sauces, Dressings, and Seasonings)

This is a very simple dish. Just mix ½ cup (4 oz) of prepackaged imitation crab with a tbs (or less) of the Sour Cream Cilantro Sauce.

Calories per Serving	Calcium (mg)	Folate (mcg)	Zinc (mg)	Fiber (g)	Protein (g)	Predicted % Omega-6
77	30	5	1	0	15	7

Overall Fat (g)	Saturated Fat (g)	Cholesterol (mg)	Short Omega-6 (mg)	Short Omega-3 (mg)	Long Omega-6 (mg)	Long Omega-3 (mg)
1	0	61	13	4	9	326

I did not find the pre-packaged imitation crab listed in the KIM-2 program, so I used the listing for three ounces of cooked pollock when calculating the nutritional data. The KIM-2 database lists three ounces of pollock at 69 calories, but the package nutritional data for Crab Delights lists a 4-oz serving as just 70 calories. Further, the KIM-2 database lists the omega-3 in three ounces of pollock as 326 mg, but the package shows only 150 mg per serving. In either case, this is a very low-calorie dish that is very low in omega-6 and very tasty.

Chicken Burrito

  1 flax tortilla (see Breads)

  ½ c roasted white meat chicken, shredded

  2 tbs tomato salsa

  2 tbs sour cream (low-fat)

  ½ c lettuce

  3 cherry tomatoes

  2 tbs chopped onion

  ½ jalapeno pepper, finely diced

  1 oz cheddar cheese, shredded

Place tortilla in a non-stick pan over medium heat and top with shredded chicken. Add salsa and cheese, fold tortilla, and cook until lightly brown. Top with lettuce, tomatoes, onion, jalapeno, and sour cream. Serve hot.

Calories per Serving	Calcium (mg)	Folate (mcg)	Zinc (mg)	Fiber (g)	Protein (g)	Predicted % Omega-6
437	302	105	3	4	35	56

Overall Fat (g)	Saturated Fat (g)	Cholesterol (mg)	Short Omega-6 (mg)	Short Omega-3 (mg)	Long Omega-6 (mg)	Long Omega-3 (mg)
20	10	105	1,294	1,128	56	42

Dinner

Seafood Dishes

Pasta in Cream Sauce with Clams and Arugula

2 c cooked pasta

1 tsp of butter

1 anchovy fillet (optional)

1 6-oz can clams

½ c arugula, chopped

½ tsp of Cajun seasoning (see Sauces, Dressings, and Seasonings)

1 clove garlic, minced

3 leaves of basil, chopped

½ c half-and-half

1 c artichoke hearts

Bring a large pot of water to a boil and cook the pasta according to package directions. Melt butter in a shallow pan and add seasoning. Pour the clams with their liquid into the pan. Chop anchovy fillet and add to pan. Bring contents to a boil, and add artichoke hearts, arugula, garlic, and basil leaves. Sauté until arugula is wilted. Add half-and-half and continue cooking until sauce is thickened. Add 2 c the cooked pasta and stir. Serves two as an entrée or four as a side dish. This recipe has 424 calories per serving as an entrée; 212 as a side dish.

Calories per Serving	Calcium (mg)	Folate (mcg)	Zinc (mg)	Fiber (g)	Protein (g)	Predicted % Omega-6
212	82	70	2	1	15	30

Overall Fat (g)	Saturated Fat (g)	Cholesterol (mg)	Short Omega-6 (mg)	Short Omega-3 (mg)	Long Omega-6 (mg)	Long Omega-3 (mg)
6	3	42	295	104	35	165

Shrimp Pasta with Cream Sauce

1 c dry, enriched egg noodle

2 tsp butter

2 cloves minced garlic

1 tbs chopped shallots

1 tbs chopped green pepper

½ tsp dried thyme

½ tsp dried basil

¼ tsp ground red pepper

2 dozen shrimp, medium (about ½ pound)

½ tsp ground white pepper

½ c artichoke hearts, drained

½ c half-and-half

Cook and drain egg noodles; set aside. Melt butter over low heat; add garlic, shallot, and green pepper, and sauté over medium-high heat until soft, 1-2 minutes. Add spices (thyme, basil, white pepper, and red pepper). Add shrimp and artichoke hearts, and sauté until shrimp are pink. Add noodles and half-and-half, simmering until the sauce thickens. Serve hot. Serves two.

Calories per Serving	Calcium (mg)	Folate (mcg)	Zinc (mg)	Fiber (g)	Protein (g)	Predicted % Omega-6
356	174	75	2	3	32	28

Overall Fat (g)	Saturated Fat (g)	Cholesterol (mg)	Short Omega-6 (mg)	Short Omega-3 (mg)	Long Omega-6 (mg)	Long Omega-3 (mg)
14	7	245	548	212	111	671

Shrimp, Crab, and Andouille Gumbo

Seasoning mix:

    1 tsp salt

    ¾ tsp red pepper

    2 bay leaves

    ½ tsp white pepper

    ½ tsp black pepper

    ½ tsp dried thyme

    ½ tsp dried oregano

Gumbo:

    ¼ c clarified butter (ghee)

    ½ c flour

    1½ c chopped onions

    1 c chopped bell pepper

    1 c chopped celery

    2 tsp minced garlic

    1 c chopped okra

    4 c seafood stock

    1 pound peeled shrimp

    1 cup crab fingers (crab claws with shell removed)

    ½ pound white fish, such as grouper, cut in 1-inch cubes

    ½ pound andouille or kielbasa sausage sliced ¼ inch thick

    Cooked rice

Prepare enough rice for a ¼-cup serving per person. Bring the seafood stock to a boil in a large pot. Then begin making a roux—the key to a good gumbo. To make the roux, put the clarified butter in a large pan and bring to high heat. When the butter is hot, stir in the flour and continue cooking and stirring until the mixture develops a rich, dark-brown color—just short of burning. When the roux is ready, add the vegetables and seasoning mix, remove from heat, and continue stirring until the vegetables stop cooking. When the stock boils, slowly add the vegetable mixture, stirring until the gumbo is the desired thickness. Add the sausage and simmer for 20 minutes. Add the shrimp and crab claws and cook a few minutes, until the shrimp are pink. Serve over rice. Serves six; 472 calories per serving.

Calories per Serving	Calcium (mg)	Folate (mcg)	Zinc (mg)	Fiber (g)	Protein (g)	Predicted % Omega-6
472	117	123	3	3	41	34

Overall Fat (g)	Saturated Fat (g)	Cholesterol (mg)	Short Omega-6 (mg)	Short Omega-3 (mg)	Long Omega-6 (mg)	Long Omega-3 (mg)
22	10	199	1,433	307	122	761

This gumbo can be made even lower in calories, fat, and omega-6. Paul Prudhomme's sister, Enola Prudhomme, has a low-calorie Cajun cookbook that uses a fat-free roux, made by simply browning flour to the color of light brown sugar. Depending on where you live, you may be able to buy dry, fat-free roux in the grocery store. If you use fat-free roux, the dish has only 286 calories. I highly recommend Enola's cookbook if you like Cajun cooking. The recipes are tasty, and you can make adjustments based on the Oil-Change Diet to make them even healthier.

Shrimp Kabobs

  1 lb shrimp, peeled and deveined

  1 c cherry tomatoes

  1 medium onion, cut in wedges

  1 green pepper, cut in large pieces (about 1-inch square)

  1 c mushrooms

  Juice of 1 lemon

  2 cloves garlic, minced

  1 tsp fresh thyme

  1 tsp paprika

  ½ tsp black pepper

  ½ tsp red pepper

  1 tsp coconut oil

Mix lemon juice, coconut oil, garlic, and spices; add shrimp and marinate for two hours in the refrigerator. Skewer shrimp and veggies together, creating repeating stacks of shrimp and each veggie, and cook on a hot grill for 8 to 10 minutes, turning frequently and basting with remaining marinade.

Calories per Serving	Calcium (mg)	Folate (mcg)	Zinc (mg)	Fiber (g)	Protein (g)	Predicted % Omega-6
140	62	25	1	2	19	31

Overall Fat (g)	Saturated Fat (g)	Cholesterol (mg)	Short Omega-6 (mg)	Short Omega-3 (mg)	Long Omega-6 (mg)	Long Omega-3 (mg)
3	1	129	231	30	74	447

Blue Crab Lollipops

1 dozen fresh, cleaned blue crabs

¼ c melted butter

1 tbs lemon juice

This dish is a fancy way to serve the best part of the blue crab. The back legs (the paddle legs) of the blue crab are prepared so that they can be broiled and eaten like a lollipop. To prepare the crab legs, cut or break the cleaned crabs in half. Lay the half crab on a cutting board and with a large knife, make a diagonal cut from the center of the crab to half way between the paddle leg and the adjacent leg. Once cut, peel the remaining shell (the white part) from the paddle leg. That should leave a nice lump of crabmeat with the paddle leg as a handle. Melt butter over low heat and add lemon juice. Place the legs on a shallow pan and drizzle them with the melted butter and lemon juice. Place the pan under a broiler and cook for 8 to 10 minutes. Arrange legs on serving plates and pour the remaining butter and lemon juice over the legs. A dozen crabs will make 2 servings of 12 legs. Save the other parts of the crabs for gumbo!

Calories per Serving	Calcium (mg)	Folate (mcg)	Zinc (mg)	Fiber (g)	Protein (g)	Predicted % Omega-6
352	158	76	6	0	31	28

Overall Fat (g)	Saturated Fat (g)	Cholesterol (mg)	Short Omega-6 (mg)	Short Omega-3 (mg)	Long Omega-6 (mg)	Long Omega-3 (mg)
25	15	195	541	335	94	544

Crab Soup

    1 c lump crab meat

    2 c half-and-half

    ¼ c green onions, chopped

    ½ tsp fresh parsley

    1 tsp butter

Sauté green onions and parsley in butter over medium-low heat. Add crabmeat and half-and-half, bring to simmer until heated through, and serve.

Calories per Serving	Calcium (mg)	Folate (mcg)	Zinc (mg)	Fiber (g)	Protein (g)	Predicted % Omega-6
439	336	51	4	0	21	29

Overall Fat (g)	Saturated Fat (g)	Cholesterol (mg)	Short Omega-6 (mg)	Short Omega-3 (mg)	Long Omega-6 (mg)	Long Omega-3 (mg)
35	21	173	788	515	57	356

Oyster Stew

    1 pt oysters

    1 tbs butter

    1 qt whole milk

    2 tbs onions, finely chopped

    ¼ c cauliflower, finely chopped

Over medium heat, sauté onions and cauliflower in butter until the onions are translucent. Add the oysters with their liquid and sauté until the oysters just start to curl at the edges. Add milk and heat to near boiling. Serve hot. Serves four.

Calories per Serving	Calcium (mg)	Folate (mcg)	Zinc (mg)	Fiber (g)	Protein (g)	Predicted % Omega-6
235	357	29	114	0	17	25

Overall Fat (g)	Saturated Fat (g)	Cholesterol (mg)	Short Omega-6 (mg)	Short Omega-3 (mg)	Long Omega-6 (mg)	Long Omega-3 (mg)
11	6	93	246	322	99	771

Using 2% milk lowers calories to 235 and does not change the percent omega-6.

Creamy Shrimp Pasta

4 tbs (½ stick) butter

1 c pasta

1 tbs minced garlic

2 tbs chopped green onion

3 tbs chopped fresh parsley

1 c sliced mushrooms

2 c half-and-half

½ tsp white pepper

½ tsp black pepper

1 c grated Parmesan cheese

1 lb shrimp, peeled and deveined

Cook the pasta until it is al dente. Meanwhile, melt the butter over medium heat, and sauté the garlic, onion, parsley, and mushrooms 2 to 3 minutes. Add half-and-half and peppers, and simmer for 5 to 6 minutes. Stir in Parmesan cheese and simmer about 5 minutes. Add shrimp and cook until pink. Stir in cooked pasta and serve. Serves four.

Calories per Serving	Calcium (mg)	Folate (mcg)	Zinc (mg)	Fiber (g)	Protein (g)	Predicted % Omega-6
601	551	79	3	1	41	27

Overall Fat (g)	Saturated Fat (g)	Cholesterol (mg)	Short Omega-6 (mg)	Short Omega-3 (mg)	Long Omega-6 (mg)	Long Omega-3 (mg)
35	21	268	876	494	99	596

Broiled Fish Parmesan

  1 firm fish fillet (such as snapper), 5 to 6 oz

  2 tsp butter

  lemon

  2 tbs fat-free sour cream

  1 tbs Parmesan cheese

  1 tsp chopped parsley

Place fish fillet in shallow pan, top with butter and two slices of lemon (cut crossways to make rounds). Broil fish until flaky. Mix sour cream, Parmesan cheese, and chopped parsley. Coat fish with sour cream mixture and return to broiler. Cook until cheese starts to brown.

Calories per Serving	Calcium (mg)	Folate (mcg)	Zinc (mg)	Fiber (g)	Protein (g)	Predicted % Omega-6
356	172	20	1	0	48	21

Overall Fat (g)	Saturated Fat (g)	Cholesterol (mg)	Short Omega-6 (mg)	Short Omega-3 (mg)	Long Omega-6 (mg)	Long Omega-3 (mg)
17	10	107	358	136	75	583

Smoked Fish Salad

Smoked mullet is my favorite, but any type of fish or even leftover fish from another recipe can be used to make this spread recipe. In some areas, mullet can have an unpleasant "muddy" flavor and is considered baitfish, but here along the central Gulf Coast, with its white sand bays, mullet is a popular fish for smoking. I smoke my own mullet and use it for this recipe often, but smoking fish is also a good way to use any strongly flavored fish, like bluefish or mackerel. You can add whatever fresh veggies you like as well as other flavorings.

1 lb of mullet, smoked, picked free of bones

1 med onion, finely chopped

1 bell pepper, finely chopped

1 c celery, finely chopped

2 jalapeno peppers, finely chopped

2 tbs hot sauce

2 tbs lemon juice, cider vinegar, or hot pepper vinegar

¼ c reduced-fat sour cream

¼ c fat-free Greek yogurt

¼ c cream cheese

¼ c pickle relish

1 tsp minced garlic

Salt and pepper to taste

Place all ingredients in a large bowl and mix thoroughly. Refrigerate. Spread on crackers for a snack or serve on a bed of lettuce as an entree. Divided into 4 portions, this dish has 217 calories per serving.

Calories per Serving	Calcium (mg)	Folate (mcg)	Zinc (mg)	Fiber (g)	Protein (g)	Predicted % Omega-6
356	172	20	1	0	48	21

Overall Fat (g)	Saturated Fat (g)	Cholesterol (mg)	Short Omega-6 (mg)	Short Omega-3 (mg)	Long Omega-6 (mg)	Long Omega-3 (mg)
17	10	107	358	136	75	583

Fish Poached in White Wine

    8 oz fish fillet

    1 c white wine

    1 tbs butter

    1 tsp minced garlic

    1 tbs chopped fresh dill

    1 tbs chopped green onions

    2 tsp dill butter (See Sauces, Dressings, and Seasonings)

Sauté garlic, dill, and onions in butter for 1 to 2 minutes over medium heat, add wine and reduce heat to a slow simmer. Add fish and simmer until the fish flakes easily. Remove fish from pan and top with dill butter. Serve hot.

Calories per Serving	Calcium (mg)	Folate (mcg)	Zinc (mg)	Fiber (g)	Protein (g)	Predicted % Omega-6
283	62	22	1	0	26	20

Overall Fat (g)	Saturated Fat (g)	Cholesterol (mg)	Short Omega-6 (mg)	Short Omega-3 (mg)	Long Omega-6 (mg)	Long Omega-3 (mg)
11	6	74	251	157	43	333

Shrimp Diane with Pasta

1 c sliced mushrooms

½ stick of butter

½ pound of shrimp, peeled and deveined (reserve shells)

¼ c chopped green onions

1 tsp minced garlic

½ tsp white pepper

½ tsp black pepper

1 tbs chopped fresh parsley

1 c cooked spaghetti

Cook the spaghetti according to package directions. Put the shrimp shells in a small pot, cover with water (about 1 to 2 cups), bring to a boil, and boil over medium-low heat for at least ten minutes. Add more water if needed so that you will end up with at least ¼ c of stock. Strain the finished stock. Reserve ¼ c for this recipe; keep any remaining stock in the freezer for adding to soups our sauces where you want shellfish flavor.

Melt the butter in a skillet over medium-high heat, add the shrimp, garlic, green onions, and peppers, and sauté until shrimp are just pink. Add mushrooms, stock, and parsley, and sauté for another couple minutes. Shaking the pan will help make an emulsion of the liquid. Serve hot over spaghetti. Serves two.

Calories per Serving	Calcium (mg)	Folate (mcg)	Zinc (mg)	Fiber (g)	Protein (g)	Predicted % Omega-6
445	94	82	2	2	29	29

Overall Fat (g)	Saturated Fat (g)	Cholesterol (mg)	Short Omega-6 (mg)	Short Omega-3 (mg)	Long Omega-6 (mg)	Long Omega-3 (mg)
26	15	234	794	378	102	624

Stuffed Flounder

6 flounder fillets, 3 to 4 oz each

12 medium shrimp

½ c chopped green pepper

½ c chopped onion

¼ c chopped celery

1 tsp Cajun seasoning

½ tsp salt

4 tbs butter

3 tbs flour

To make the stuffing, melt 1 tbs of butter over medium heat and sauté the green pepper, onion, and celery until the onions start to brown. Add shrimp and Cajun seasoning and cook until shrimp are pink. Puree the shrimp and vegetables in a blender. Melt 2 tbs of butter over medium-low heat, add 2 tbs of flour and stir. Add blended shrimp and cook until mixture starts to stick together. Divide the stuffing mixture evenly among the fish fillets, then roll up each fillet and secure it with a toothpick. Coat rolls lightly with the remaining tbs of flour and cook them in a non-stick pan with the remaining butter until lightly brown on each side. Serves six.

Calories per Serving	Calcium (mg)	Folate (mcg)	Zinc (mg)	Fiber (g)	Protein (g)	Predicted % Omega-6
188	31	24	1	1	20	25

Overall Fat (g)	Saturated Fat (g)	Cholesterol (mg)	Short Omega-6 (mg)	Short Omega-3 (mg)	Long Omega-6 (mg)	Long Omega-3 (mg)
9	5	83	227	138	44	282

Jambalaya with Shrimp and Sausage

Seasoning Mix:

   1 tsp red pepper

   1 tsp paprika

   1 tsp white pepper

   1 tsp mustard

   1 tsp salt

   1 tsp gumbo filé powder

   2 bay leaves

   ½ tsp black pepper

   ½ tsp cumin

   ½ tsp thyme leaves

Jambalaya:

   2 tbs butter

   1 c chopped onion

   1 c chopped celery

   1 c chopped bell pepper

   ½ tbs minced garlic

   2 c rice

   4 c stock

   1 c chopped tomatoes

   ½ pound shrimp, peeled

   3 oz andouille or kielbasa sausage

Melt butter over medium heat; add veggies, seasoning mix, and sausage, and sauté until onions are caramelized, stirring and scraping the pan bottom. Add rice and continue stirring a couple minutes. Add stock and simmer until about the liquid is reduced by half (about 7 minutes). Add shrimp and cook until rice is tender (about 7 more minutes). Serves four.

Calories per Serving	Calcium (mg)	Folate (mcg)	Zinc (mg)	Fiber (g)	Protein (g)	Predicted % Omega-6
631	99	308	3	5	30	28

Overall Fat (g)	Saturated Fat (g)	Cholesterol (mg)	Short Omega-6 (mg)	Short Omega-3 (mg)	Long Omega-6 (mg)	Long Omega-3 (mg)
16	7	130	1,137	248	81	571

Spinach and Artichoke Pasta with Crab

    1 tsp butter

    1 can crab meat (6.5 oz)

    · 1 c elbow macaroni, dry

    ½ c artichoke hearts, drained

    1 c spinach, cooked and drained

    1 c half-and-half

Cook macaroni according to package directions. Check canned crab for any pieces of shell. Melt butter in a saucepan, add all other ingredients, mix and heat thoroughly. Serves four.

Calories per Serving	Calcium (mg)	Folate (mcg)	Zinc (mg)	Fiber (g)	Protein (g)	Predicted % Omega-6
237	171	152	2	3	14	30

Overall Fat (g)	Saturated Fat (g)	Cholesterol (mg)	Short Omega-6 (mg)	Short Omega-3 (mg)	Long Omega-6 (mg)	Long Omega-3 (mg)
9	5	53	357	173	20	113

Stir-Fried Shrimp

  1 tbs coconut oil

  1 c shredded cabbage

  ½ c chopped arugula

  ½ c chopped onion

  ½ c snow peas

  6 oz shrimp

  ½ c rice

Cook rice. Sauté veggies and shrimp in oil over medium heat until veggies are tender and shrimp are pink. Serve over rice. Serves two.

Calories per Serving	Calcium (mg)	Folate (mcg)	Zinc (mg)	Fiber (g)	Protein (g)	Predicted % Omega-6
269	107	114	2	5	23	23

Overall Fat (g)	Saturated Fat (g)	Cholesterol (mg)	Short Omega-6 (mg)	Short Omega-3 (mg)	Long Omega-6 (mg)	Long Omega-3 (mg)
2	0	129	167	66	74	447

This recipe, like all stir-fry recipes, is very versatile. A wide variety of veggies can be used, including green and red peppers, broccoli, artichoke hearts, celery, bok choy, carrots, bamboo shoots, water chestnuts, or bean sprouts. You can also use noodles instead of rice, including the zero-calorie shirataki noodles. A variety of different sauces can be added to change the flavor as well.

Shrimp Creole

    2 tbs butter

    1 lb shrimp, peeled and deveined

    Creole Sauce (see Sauces, Dressings, and Seasonings)

    ½ c long-grain rice

Cook rice. Melt butter in a pan over medium heat and sauté shrimp until pink. Add creole sauce and simmer 2 to 3 minutes. Serve hot over rice. Serves four.

Calories per Serving	Calcium (mg)	Folate (mcg)	Zinc (mg)	Fiber (g)	Protein (g)	Predicted % Omega-6
359	105	63	2	3	26	30

Overall Fat (g)	Saturated Fat (g)	Cholesterol (mg)	Short Omega-6 (mg)	Short Omega-3 (mg)	Long Omega-6 (mg)	Long Omega-3 (mg)
17	9	211	683	271	98	595

Mussels in Wine Sauce

1 lb fresh mussels

3 tbs butter

1 c white wine

¼ c chopped green onions

2 tsp minced garlic

1 tsp fresh thyme

¼ tsp salt

¼ tsp black pepper

Scrub and de-beard the mussels. Discard any that do not close when touched. Add all ingredients to a large pot and bring to a boil. Cook for about 5 minutes, stirring occasionally. When most of the mussels are open, remove them with a slotted spoon and place into 2 serving bowls. Discard any mussels that did not open. Continue cooking the sauce for about 5 minutes. Pour wine sauce over mussels and serve. Serves two.

Calories per Serving	Calcium (mg)	Folate (mcg)	Zinc (mg)	Fiber (g)	Protein (g)	Predicted % Omega-6
437	96	103	4	0	28	26

Overall Fat (g)	Saturated Fat (g)	Cholesterol (mg)	Short Omega-6 (mg)	Short Omega-3 (mg)	Long Omega-6 (mg)	Long Omega-3 (mg)
22	12	110	450	380	158	1,042

Fish with Mango Salsa

    1 red snapper fillet (about 8 oz)

    1 tsp butter

    1 c Mango Salsa (see Sauces, Dressings, and Seasonings)

    ½ c rice

Cook rice. Melt butter over medium heat in a non-stick pan. Sauté fish over medium heat until almost done (firm in the center but flaky only at the edges, about 4–5 minutes per side). Add mango salsa and sauté for 2–3 minutes or until salsa is warm and fish is done through (flakes when tested in the center with a fork, or reaches 145° on a thermometer inserted into the center of the thickest part of the fillet). Serve over rice. Serves two.

Calories per Serving	Calcium (mg)	Folate (mcg)	Zinc (mg)	Fiber (g)	Protein (g)	Predicted % Omega-6
171	46	20	0	1	23	22

Overall Fat (g)	Saturated Fat (g)	Cholesterol (mg)	Short Omega-6 (mg)	Short Omega-3 (mg)	Long Omega-6 (mg)	Long Omega-3 (mg)
4	2	45	100	65	53	410

Shrimp with Mango Salsa

½ lb shrimp, peeled and deveined

1 tsp coconut oil

1 c Mango Salsa (see Sauces)

½ c rice

Cook rice. Sauté shrimp in coconut oil over medium heat until just pink. Add mango salsa and continue cooking for 2 to 3 minutes, until shrimp are pink and salsa is heated through. Serve over a bed of rice or pasta. Serves two.

Calories per Serving	Calcium (mg)	Folate (mcg)	Zinc (mg)	Fiber (g)	Protein (g)	Predicted % Omega-6
354	143	22	3	1	52	29

Overall Fat (g)	Saturated Fat (g)	Cholesterol (mg)	Short Omega-6 (mg)	Short Omega-3 (mg)	Long Omega-6 (mg)	Long Omega-3 (mg)
9	5	388	189	74	222	1,341

Low-Country Boil

This is one of my favorite recipes for large gatherings of family or friends. It is a one-pot dish that provides a complete meal. I like to use head-on shrimp and allow a half-pound per person. If you use head-on shrimp, make sure they are fresh, with heads firmly attached and without lots of orange color in the heads.

Shrimp, ½ lb per person

Potatoes, 1 per person

Corn on the cob, 1 half ear per person

Sausage, 1 4-inch link per person

1 lemon, halved, for every 5 pounds of shrimp

2 onions, halved, for every 5 pounds of shrimp

1 bulb garlic, halved, for every 5 pounds of shrimp

1 stalk celery for every 5 pounds of shrimp

Seasoning: Use one mesh bag of crab and shrimp boil plus a half pound of a granular seasoning mix, like Zatarain's or Louisiana, for every 5 pounds of shrimp

Place potatoes, lemons, onions, garlic, celery, and seasonings in a large pot, add enough water to cover, and boil until potatoes are almost done. Add shrimp, corn, and sausage, and bring back to a boil. Turn off heat as soon as the pot reaches a boil. Let everything stand in the hot water for about 10 to 15 minutes, until the shrimp are done. Test a few shrimp as they soak to make sure they are not getting over-cooked (over-cooked shrimp are hard to shell). Serve hot. One serving includes a half-pound of shrimp, a potato, a piece of corn, and a sausage link.

Calories per Serving	Calcium (mg)	Folate (mcg)	Zinc (mg)	Fiber (g)	Protein (g)	Predicted % Omega-6
413	87	56	3	4	35	38

Overall Fat (g)	Saturated Fat (g)	Cholesterol (mg)	Short Omega-6 (mg)	Short Omega-3 (mg)	Long Omega-6 (mg)	Long Omega-3 (mg)
14	4	195	1,503	179	98	595

Poultry Dishes

Chicken Florentine

　　8 oz boneless, skinless chicken breasts, cut in strips

　　10 oz package chopped, frozen spinach, cooked and drained

　　2 tbs butter

　　2 tbs flour

　　½ tsp salt

　　1 c half-and-half

　　¼ c Parmesan cheese

　　Salt and pepper or seasoning mix to taste

Season chicken pieces and sauté over medium heat in a tablespoon of butter until lightly brown. Remove chicken and set aside. Melt the remaining butter, whisk in the flour, and add the spinach and half-and-half. Simmer until thickened, then add Parmesan cheese and return chicken to pan. Simmer for an additional 2 to 3 minutes. Serve over pasta or rice. Serves two.

Calories per Serving	Calcium (mg)	Folate (mcg)	Zinc (mg)	Fiber (g)	Protein (g)	Predicted % Omega-6
537	475	210	3	5	42	53

Overall Fat (g)	Saturated Fat (g)	Cholesterol (mg)	Short Omega-6 (mg)	Short Omega-3 (mg)	Long Omega-6 (mg)	Long Omega-3 (mg)
31	19	154	904	574	47	35

Calorie amount does not include rice or pasta.

Mushroom Chicken with Mashed Potatoes

1 tsp coconut oil or butter

½ boneless, skinless chicken breast

8 oz mushrooms

½ c chopped onion

¼ c chopped green onion

1 c chicken broth

1 tbs cornstarch

¾ tsp paprika

½ tsp white pepper

½ tsp black pepper

½ tsp garlic powder

½ tsp salt

1 c mashed potatoes

Cut chicken breast into strips and brown over medium heat in coconut oil or butter. Add mushrooms, onions, and spices, and continue cooking until onions are tender. Mix cornstarch with broth and add to chicken. Simmer for 20 to 30 minutes. Serve over ½ cup of mashed potatoes. Serves two.

Calories per Serving	Calcium (mg)	Folate (mcg)	Zinc (mg)	Fiber (g)	Protein (g)	Predicted % Omega-6
256	45	17	1	3	18	58

Overall Fat (g)	Saturated Fat (g)	Cholesterol (mg)	Short Omega-6 (mg)	Short Omega-3 (mg)	Long Omega-6 (mg)	Long Omega-3 (mg)
4	3	36	321	36	24	18

Chicken Broccoli Cheese Casserole

1 c chopped roasted chicken (white meat)

2 c chopped cooked broccoli

½ c shredded cheddar cheese

½ c liquid eggs (fat-free)

½ c half-and-half

¼ c milled flax seed

¼ c Parmesan cheese

Salt and pepper to taste

Place broccoli in casserole dish and top with chicken. Mix cheddar cheese, half-and-half, egg whites, and milled flax seed, and pour over chicken and broccoli. Sprinkle with Parmesan cheese and bake at 350° for about 30 minutes. Serves four.

Calories per Serving	Calcium (mg)	Folate (mcg)	Zinc (mg)	Fiber (g)	Protein (g)	Predicted % Omega-6
447	310	111	3	2	35	59

Overall Fat (g)	Saturated Fat (g)	Cholesterol (mg)	Short Omega-6 (mg)	Short Omega-3 (mg)	Long Omega-6 (mg)	Long Omega-3 (mg)
19	11	112	797	319	42	28

Chicken Tortilla Casserole

    2 c roasted white-meat chicken, chopped

    2 c shredded cheddar cheese

    2 c canned diced tomatoes

    ½ c half-and-half

    2 flax tortillas, torn into pieces (see Breads)

    1 tbs hot pepper sauce

    1 small can green chiles, diced

    1 c fat-free sour cream

    ¼ c milled flax seed

Mix chicken, tomatoes, cream, pepper sauce, green chiles, sour cream, and flax seed in a bowl. Put about 1/3 of the mixture into a casserole dish, add a layer of flax tortilla pieces, and then a layer of cheddar cheese. Repeat layers two more times. Bake at 375° for 30 minutes. If cheese starts to brown too much, cover with foil and continue cooking. Serves four.

Calories per Serving	Calcium (mg)	Folate (mcg)	Zinc (mg)	Fiber (g)	Protein (g)	Predicted % Omega-6
583	461	95	3	6	40	48

Overall Fat (g)	Saturated Fat (g)	Cholesterol (mg)	Short Omega-6 (mg)	Short Omega-3 (mg)	Long Omega-6 (mg)	Long Omega-3 (mg)
35	18	145	1,951	2,583	42	28

Stir-Fried Chicken

4 oz boneless, skinless chicken breast, sliced into ½-inch chunks

1 tbs of oil

1 c shredded cabbage

1 c broccoli florets

1 c cauliflower, sliced

½ c chopped onion

½ c snow peas

1 c cooked rice

½ c chicken broth

1 tbs of cornstarch

Sauté chicken in coconut oil over medium heat until lightly browned. Add veggies and cook until fork-tender. In a separate pan, add cornstarch to cold chicken broth, heat until sauce thickens, and add to chicken and veggies. Add rice and cook until rice is hot. Serves two.

Calories per Serving	Calcium (mg)	Folate (mcg)	Zinc (mg)	Fiber (g)	Protein (g)	Predicted % Omega-6
367	75	145	1	4	19	57

Overall Fat (g)	Saturated Fat (g)	Cholesterol (mg)	Short Omega-6 (mg)	Short Omega-3 (mg)	Long Omega-6 (mg)	Long Omega-3 (mg)
11	7	26	736	1,219	27	18

With ½ tbs milled flax seed per serving added after cooking:

Calories per Serving	Calcium (mg)	Folate (mcg)	Zinc (mg)	Fiber (g)	Protein (g)	Predicted % Omega-6
396	87	162	2	6	20	42

Overall Fat (g)	Saturated Fat (g)	Cholesterol (mg)	Short Omega-6 (mg)	Short Omega-3 (mg)	Long Omega-6 (mg)	Long Omega-3 (mg)
11	7	26	736	1,219	27	18

Meat Dishes

Chili with Beans

- ½ lb ground venison
- 1 medium onion, chopped
- 1 16-oz can whole tomatoes
- 1 16-oz can pinto beans
- 1 tsp minced garlic
- 3 tbs chili powder
- 1 tbs paprika
- 1 tbs cumin
- 1 tsp cayenne pepper
- 1 tsp sea salt

Brown meat over medium-high heat with the onions and garlic. Add tomatoes, beans, and spices. Simmer for 30 minutes. Serves four.

Calories per Serving	Calcium (mg)	Folate (mcg)	Zinc (mg)	Fiber (g)	Protein (g)	Predicted % Omega-6
249	120	172	3	12	23	88

Overall Fat (g)	Saturated Fat (g)	Cholesterol (mg)	Short Omega-6 (mg)	Short Omega-3 (mg)	Long Omega-6 (mg)	Long Omega-3 (mg)
4	1	48	909	199	57	0

Adding a tbs of milled flax seed to each serving will reduce omega-6 to 57 percent.

Burrito Supreme

1 10-inch flour tortilla

3 oz ground beef

¼ c black beans, drained

1 oz cheddar cheese, shredded

¼ c chopped onions

1 c chopped lettuce

1 tbs sour cream

1 jalapeno pepper, chopped

1 tsp cumin

1 tsp chili powder

1 tsp paprika

1 tsp cayenne pepper

Brown the ground beef over medium heat with the spices. Add the beans and simmer until heated through. Place meat and bean mixture on a tortilla with half of the cheese. Fold into a burrito and top with lettuce, tomatoes, onions, jalapeno, the remaining cheese, and sour cream.

Calories per Serving	Calcium (mg)	Folate (mcg)	Zinc (mg)	Fiber (g)	Protein (g)	Predicted % Omega-6
545	303	227	8	10	40	57

Overall Fat (g)	Saturated Fat (g)	Cholesterol (mg)	Short Omega-6 (mg)	Short Omega-3 (mg)	Long Omega-6 (mg)	Long Omega-3 (mg)
25	15	98	1,370	1,189	43	0

Contains 628 calories and produces 74 percent long omega-6. With 1 tbs of milled flax seed, the long omega-6 drops to 53 percent and calories increase to 687. If you use a flax tortilla (see Breads) instead of a commercial flour tortilla, the burrito has just 545 calories and 57 percent long omega-6.

Stir-Fried Pork

　　1 tbs coconut oil

　　1 c chopped cabbage

　　½ c chopped broccoli

　　½ c carrots, julienned

　　½ c chopped onions

　　½ c snow peas

　　3 oz lean pork, thinly sliced

　　1 c cooked rice

Sauté veggies and pork in oil over medium heat until the vegetable are fork-tender. Add cooked rice and stir until fully heated. Serves two.

Calories per Serving	Calcium (mg)	Folate (mcg)	Zinc (mg)	Fiber (g)	Protein (g)	Predicted % Omega-6
411	59	161	2	4	16	69

Overall Fat (g)	Saturated Fat (g)	Cholesterol (mg)	Short Omega-6 (mg)	Short Omega-3 (mg)	Long Omega-6 (mg)	Long Omega-3 (mg)
10	7	26	498	84	30	0

With a tablespoon of milled flax seed added to each serving:

Calories per Serving	Calcium (mg)	Folate (mcg)	Zinc (mg)	Fiber (g)	Protein (g)	Predicted % Omega-6
470	83	194	2	7	18	39

Overall Fat (g)	Saturated Fat (g)	Cholesterol (mg)	Short Omega-6 (mg)	Short Omega-3 (mg)	Long Omega-6 (mg)	Long Omega-3 (mg)
14	7	26	1,016	2,258	30	0

Vegetarian Entrées and Sides

Fresh Fruit Salad

1 nectarine, chopped

1 mandarin orange, chopped

½ c blueberries

½ c strawberries, quartered

¼ c shredded coconut

¼ c chia seeds

¼ c dried cranberries

Mix all ingredients and serve. This combination of fruits works well, but use any mixture of fruits that is fresh and that inspires you. It is great over pancakes, as a side dish, or even for dessert. Serves four.

Calories per Serving	Calcium (mg)	Folate (mcg)	Zinc (mg)	Fiber (g)	Protein (g)	Predicted % Omega-6
153	85	27	1	2	3	48

Overall Fat (g)	Saturated Fat (g)	Cholesterol (mg)	Short Omega-6 (mg)	Short Omega-3 (mg)	Long Omega-6 (mg)	Long Omega-3 (mg)
7	4	0	608	579	0	0

Squash Casserole

    2 c yellow squash, boiled and drained

    2 c zucchini squash, boiled and drained

    ½ c shredded cheddar cheese

    ½ c shredded mozzarella cheese

    ½ c chopped onions

    ½ c chopped bell pepper

Combine all ingredients in layers in a casserole dish, with these cheeses as the top layer. Bake at 350° for about 30 minutes or until cheese starts to brown. Serves four.

Calories per Serving	Calcium (mg)	Folate (mcg)	Zinc (mg)	Fiber (g)	Protein (g)	Predicted % Omega-6
142	247	45	1	3	9	48

Overall Fat (g)	Saturated Fat (g)	Cholesterol (mg)	Short Omega-6 (mg)	Short Omega-3 (mg)	Long Omega-6 (mg)	Long Omega-3 (mg)
7	5	22	213	160	0	0

Eggplant Casserole

   2 c eggplant, cubed

   1 c chopped tomatoes

   1 c cheddar cheese, shredded

   1 c mozzarella cheese (part skin), shredded

   1 c crushed saltine crackers

   1 packet of onion soup mix

   ¼ c milled flax seed

Cube the eggplant and toss it with salt, then transfer the eggplant to a colander to let it drain for 30 minutes to an hour. The salt will draw out any bitterness in the eggplant. Rinse and dry the eggplant thoroughly. Sauté the eggplant in a little butter, or spread on a shallow tray and broil, stirring occasionally to encourage even cooking. When the eggplant is soft, transfer it to a casserole dish and mix in all the other ingredients except the flax seed, reserving some of the cheese for topping. Bake at 325° for 30 to 40 minutes until cheese is lightly browned. Top with flax seed and serve. Serves four.

Calories per Serving	Calcium (mg)	Folate (mcg)	Zinc (mg)	Fiber (g)	Protein (g)	Predicted % Omega-6
345	458	71	2	5	19	36

Overall Fat (g)	Saturated Fat (g)	Cholesterol (mg)	Short Omega-6 (mg)	Short Omega-3 (mg)	Long Omega-6 (mg)	Long Omega-3 (mg)
20	10	45	1,071	1,925	0	0

Sautéed Zucchini with Feta Cheese

2 c sliced zucchini squash

½ c chopped onions

½ c chopped tomatoes

½ c feta cheese

1 tsp fresh basil, chopped

1 tsp butter

Melt butter over medium heat in a non-stick pan. Add squash, onions, and tomatoes, and increase the heat to medium-high. Cook until onions are clear (squash will still be a little firm). Add feta and basil, and toss just before serving.

Calories per Serving	Calcium (mg)	Folate (mcg)	Zinc (mg)	Fiber (g)	Protein (g)	Predicted % Omega-6
79	107	26	1	1	4	51

Overall Fat (g)	Saturated Fat (g)	Cholesterol (mg)	Short Omega-6 (mg)	Short Omega-3 (mg)	Long Omega-6 (mg)	Long Omega-3 (mg)
5	3	19	138	89	0	0

Chile Relleno Casserole

  4 egg whites

  4 large green chili peppers, roasted and peeled

  4 oz mozzarella cheese

  ¼ c low-fat milk

  1 tbs flour

  1 tbs milled flax seed

In some areas, you can buy chiles already roasted. If you want to roast them yourself, simply place them under a high broiler until the skin blackens, turning them every few minutes to char all sides. You can also char them directly over the flame of a gas burner. Remove the blackened peppers to a bowl and cover with plastic wrap to steam for a few minutes. This will make the skin easy to peel off. You can rinse off any remaining char, although a little bit will enhance the flavor.

Stuff the roasted peppers with the cheese and place them in a casserole dish. Whip the egg whites until frothy, with fine bubbles and stiff peaks. Stir together the half-and-half, flax seed, and flour, and fold into the egg whites. Pour the egg mixture over the stuffed peppers and bake at 325° for 30 minutes or until golden brown. Serves four.

Calories per Serving	Calcium (mg)	Folate (mcg)	Zinc (mg)	Fiber (g)	Protein (g)	Predicted % Omega-6
82	142	30	1	1	8	30

Overall Fat (g)	Saturated Fat (g)	Cholesterol (mg)	Short Omega-6 (mg)	Short Omega-3 (mg)	Long Omega-6 (mg)	Long Omega-3 (mg)
4	2	8	232	567	0	0

Creamed Cauliflower

2 c cauliflower florets and chopped stems

1 tbs butter

¼ c half-and-half

Salt to taste

Steam or roast the cauliflower until it is very tender. Then mash or blend the cauliflower with butter and cream until smooth. Serves four.

Calories per Serving	Calcium (mg)	Folate (mcg)	Zinc (mg)	Fiber (g)	Protein (g)	Predicted % Omega-6
59	27	28	0	2	2	42

Overall Fat (g)	Saturated Fat (g)	Cholesterol (mg)	Short Omega-6 (mg)	Short Omega-3 (mg)	Long Omega-6 (mg)	Long Omega-3 (mg)
5	3	13	135	171	0	0

This recipe has just 59 calories and 42 percent omega-6. It makes a good substitute for mashed potatoes for diabetics.

Black Bean Quesadillas

    1 white onion, thinly sliced

    3 tbs butter

    1 tbs chopped garlic

    ¼ tsp cumin

    2 c cooked black beans

    2 tbs water

    1 tbs fresh cilantro, chopped

    fresh juice of half a lime

    dash hot sauce

    1 c shredded cheddar cheese

    4 flax tortillas

    salt and pepper to taste

Heat a large sauté pan on medium-high heat. Add 1 tbs of the butter and the onion. Cook for five to seven minutes until onion is caramelized. Add the garlic and cumin and cook for another minute. Add the beans, water, lime juice, hot sauce, and salt and pepper, and cook for one minute. Mash the beans with a fork to create a chunky and thick mixture. Allow the bean mixture to cool.

Spoon one quarter of the bean mixture on a tortilla and spread evenly to cover half the tortilla. Place a quarter of the shredded cheddar over the bean mixture and top with cilantro. Fold the tortilla over and gently press down. Repeat this process with the remaining tortillas.

Melt the remaining butter on medium-low heat in a large nonstick pan. Place two quesadillas at a time in the pan and cook for about two minutes on each side until crispy and golden. Drain on a paper towel. Serves four.

Calories per Serving	Calcium (mg)	Folate (mcg)	Zinc (mg)	Fiber (g)	Protein (g)	Predicted % Omega-6
350	246	154	2	9	16	45

Overall Fat (g)	Saturated Fat (g)	Cholesterol (mg)	Short Omega-6 (mg)	Short Omega-3 (mg)	Long Omega-6 (mg)	Long Omega-3 (mg)
19	12	54	576	547	0	0

Zucchini Pancakes

  2 c zucchini, shredded (see note below)

  1 egg

  1 c flour

  ¼ c milled flax seed

  ½ tsp salt

Mix zucchini, egg, flour, flax seed, and salt in a bowl. Pour about ¼ cup onto a hot non-stick pan and brown on both sides. Makes about 6 pancakes.

Calories per Serving	Calcium (mg)	Folate (mcg)	Zinc (mg)	Fiber (g)	Protein (g)	Predicted % Omega-6
86	22	48	0	3	5	24

Overall Fat (g)	Saturated Fat (g)	Cholesterol (mg)	Short Omega-6 (mg)	Short Omega-3 (mg)	Long Omega-6 (mg)	Long Omega-3 (mg)
2	0	0	329	1,188	0	0

Each pancake has 126 calories and 40 percent long omega-6.

If you use frozen zucchini, be sure to let it thaw and drain before using. If you are using fresh zucchini, salt it, let it sit 30 minutes, and then squeeze it to express most of its water content.

Skeet Taters

Skeet is my nickname, and my buddies at our duck camp named this recipe after me. They love it and expect it on every trip.

  2 sweet potatoes, peeled and cut into irregular fries

  1 tbs coconut oil

  garlic salt to taste

Spread fries on a baking sheet; drizzle with the coconut oil and sprinkle with garlic salt. Bake at 400° until potato slices are starting to brown along the edges (about 20 to 25 minutes). Serves four.

Calories per Serving	Calcium (mg)	Folate (mcg)	Zinc (mg)	Fiber (g)	Protein (g)	Predicted % Omega-6
101	15	9	0	2	1	63

Overall Fat (g)	Saturated Fat (g)	Cholesterol (mg)	Short Omega-6 (mg)	Short Omega-3 (mg)	Long Omega-6 (mg)	Long Omega-3 (mg)
4	3	0	137	14	0	0

Roasted Butternut Squash

1 medium butternut squash, peeled and cut into ¼- to ½-inch strips

1 tsp butter

garlic salt

Spread softened butter over squash and toss to get some of the butter on each of the pieces. Sprinkle with garlic salt and roast in oven at 400° for about 20 to 25 minutes or until the squash is starting to brown. Serves four.

Calories per Serving	Calcium (mg)	Folate (mcg)	Zinc (mg)	Fiber (g)	Protein (g)	Predicted % Omega-6
80	68	38	0	0	1	41

Overall Fat (g)	Saturated Fat (g)	Cholesterol (mg)	Short Omega-6 (mg)	Short Omega-3 (mg)	Long Omega-6 (mg)	Long Omega-3 (mg)
2	1	5	65	64	0	0

Broccoli Cheese Casserole

2 c broccoli, chopped

1 c liquid eggs (fat-free)

1 c cheddar cheese

½ c long-grain rice

Cook the rice. Meanwhile, steam the broccoli until it is tender but still firm. Put cooked rice in a casserole dish, top with broccoli, pour in liquid eggs, and top with cheese. Bake at 350° for about 30 minutes. Serves four.

Calories per Serving	Calcium (mg)	Folate (mcg)	Zinc (mg)	Fiber (g)	Protein (g)	Predicted % Omega-6
216	252	79	1	2	17	43

Overall Fat (g)	Saturated Fat (g)	Cholesterol (mg)	Short Omega-6 (mg)	Short Omega-3 (mg)	Long Omega-6 (mg)	Long Omega-3 (mg)
10	6	30	218	209	0	0

Red Cabbage with Apples

1 medium red cabbage, shredded

1 large apple, thinly sliced

½ c red wine vinegar

½ c red wine

½ c brown sugar

1 tbs butter

2 tbs flour

Steam the cabbage until tender but still firm. Melt the butter in a saucepan, add the flour, and stir 1 minute. Add the vinegar, wine, and brown sugar. Bring to a boil, pour over steamed cabbage, add apple slices, and mix. Makes 6 servings.

Calories per Serving	Calcium (mg)	Folate (mcg)	Zinc (mg)	Fiber (g)	Protein (g)	Predicted % Omega-6
155	66	32	0	3	2	47

Overall Fat (g)	Saturated Fat (g)	Cholesterol (mg)	Short Omega-6 (mg)	Short Omega-3 (mg)	Long Omega-6 (mg)	Long Omega-3 (mg)
2	1	5	143	99	0	0

Vegetable Chili

 1 16-oz can pinto beans

 1 16-oz can diced tomatoes

 1 c chopped onion

 1 16-oz can black beans

 1 c hominy

 1 tbs minced garlic

 3 tbs chili powder

 1 tbs cumin

 1 tsp red pepper

 1 tsp paprika

 1 tsp salt

 1 tbs milled flax seed

Mix all ingredients except flax seed and simmer for 20 to 30 minutes to allow flavors to marry. Add flax seed and serve. Serves six.

Calories per Serving	Calcium (mg)	Folate (mcg)	Zinc (mg)	Fiber (g)	Protein (g)	Predicted % Omega-6
176	74	131	1	11	9	51

Overall Fat (g)	Saturated Fat (g)	Cholesterol (mg)	Short Omega-6 (mg)	Short Omega-3 (mg)	Long Omega-6 (mg)	Long Omega-3 (mg)
2	0	0	643	512	0	0

Black Bean Corn Salsa

1 16-oz can black beans

1 16-oz can diced tomatoes

1 c white shoe peg corn

½ c chopped onions

1 tbs chopped fresh cilantro

1 tsp cumin

1 tsp minced garlic

1 tsp black pepper

1 tsp salt

Combine all ingredients and serve. This can work as a main-dish salad or as a side. As a main dish, it serves two.

Calories per Serving	Calcium (mg)	Folate (mcg)	Zinc (mg)	Fiber (g)	Protein (g)	Predicted % Omega-6
381	119	338	3	21	21	39

Overall Fat (g)	Saturated Fat (g)	Cholesterol (mg)	Short Omega-6 (mg)	Short Omega-3 (mg)	Long Omega-6 (mg)	Long Omega-3 (mg)
4	1	0	885	1,284	0	0

With just a teaspoon of flax seed, the omega-6 is 49 percent. With a tablespoon of flax seed, the omega-6 drops to 39 percent. Without flax seed it is 351 calories and 59 percent omega-6.

Eggplant Lasagna

  2 c eggplant diced, cooked and drained

  1 package Lipton onion soup mix

  1 16-oz can diced tomatoes

  1 tbs milled flax seed

  1 tsp basil

  1 tsp oregano

  ½ tsp thyme

  1 c ricotta cheese (part skim)

  1 c cottage cheese (fat-free)

  8 oz package of lasagna noodles

  salt to taste

  ¼ c Parmesan cheese

Mix eggplant, soup mix, tomatoes, flax seed, and spices in a bowl. Combine the ricotta and cottage cheese. Layer eggplant mixture, lasagna noodles, and cheese mixture in a casserole dish to create 3 or 4 layers of each ingredient. Top with the Parmesan cheese and bake at 350° for about 25 minutes. Serves four.

Calories per Serving	Calcium (mg)	Folate (mcg)	Zinc (mg)	Fiber (g)	Protein (g)	Predicted % Omega-6
392	340	160	2	5	25	45

Overall Fat (g)	Saturated Fat (g)	Cholesterol (mg)	Short Omega-6 (mg)	Short Omega-3 (mg)	Long Omega-6 (mg)	Long Omega-3 (mg)
9	5	27	682	668	0	0

KIM-2 does not have data on lasagna noodles; I used the numbers for 8 oz of macaroni. Without the flax seed, this dish is 60 percent omega-6.

Red Beans and Rice

Red beans and rice is a staple in New Orleans. It is a simple dish usually served on Mondays to make up for the excesses of the weekend. We try to have a meal of legumes at least once a week.

1 c dried red kidney beans

¼ c chopped onions

¼ c chopped celery

1 bay leaf

½ c cooked rice

2 oz lean ham

Cover beans in 1 quart of water and soak overnight. Pour off the water and rinse the beans before cooking. Put the beans in a crock-pot pot with the onions, celery, and spices, and add enough water to cover by 2 to 3 inches. Cook on high for 4 to 8 hours. Serve over cooked rice. Serves four.

Calories per Serving	Calcium (mg)	Folate (mcg)	Zinc (mg)	Fiber (g)	Protein (g)	Predicted % Omega-6
209	47	200	2	7	14	42

Overall Fat (g)	Saturated Fat (g)	Cholesterol (mg)	Short Omega-6 (mg)	Short Omega-3 (mg)	Long Omega-6 (mg)	Long Omega-3 (mg)
1	0	5	181	173	0	0

Baked Potato with Cheese, Sour Cream, and Flax Seed

A typical large baked potato dressed with an ounce of reduced-fat sour cream and cheddar cheese is not a bad choice on its own, with just 433 calories and 48 percent omega-6; however, with just a teaspoon of milled flax seed, it drops to 35 percent omega-6.

Calories per Serving	Calcium (mg)	Folate (mcg)	Zinc (mg)	Fiber (g)	Protein (g)	Predicted % Omega-6
452	288	103	2	8	16	35

Overall Fat (g)	Saturated Fat (g)	Cholesterol (mg)	Short Omega-6 (mg)	Short Omega-3 (mg)	Long Omega-6 (mg)	Long Omega-3 (mg)
15	8	41	544	912	0	0

Sauces, Dressings, and Seasonings

Flax Mayonnaise

    1½ c coconut oil

    1 large egg

    1 tbs of vinegar

    1 tsp salt

    ½ tsp white pepper

    ¼ c milled flax seed

Place egg in blender and blend for about 30 seconds. With blender on, add coconut oil in a steady stream, continuing to blend until it is thick and creamy. Add vinegar and blend for another 30 seconds. Add flax seed, salt, and pepper, and blend for about 1 minute.

Calories per Serving	Calcium (mg)	Folate (mcg)	Zinc (mg)	Fiber (g)	Protein (g)	Predicted % Omega-6
97	3	4	0	0	0	51

Overall Fat (g)	Saturated Fat (g)	Cholesterol (mg)	Short Omega-6 (mg)	Short Omega-3 (mg)	Long Omega-6 (mg)	Long Omega-3 (mg)
11	9	7	254	220	2	1

Sour Cream and Yogurt Hot Sauce

¼ c fat-free Greek yogurt

¼ c fat-free sour cream

¼ c skim milk

1 tbs of hot sauce (such as Tabasco)

Mix all ingredients in a saucepan and simmer until hot. This sauce is great over roasted chicken or turkey. It can also be used in place of mayonnaise on sandwiches. Serves two.

Calories per Serving	Calcium (mg)	Folate (mcg)	Zinc (mg)	Fiber (g)	Protein (g)	Predicted % Omega-6
71	137	9	1	0	4	52

Overall Fat (g)	Saturated Fat (g)	Cholesterol (mg)	Short Omega-6 (mg)	Short Omega-3 (mg)	Long Omega-6 (mg)	Long Omega-3 (mg)
4	2	13	99	54	0	0

Creole Sauce

- 2 bay leaves
- ¾ tsp oregano
- ½ tsp salt
- ½ tsp white pepper
- ½ tsp black pepper
- ½ tsp red pepper
- ½ tsp paprika
- ½ tsp basil
- 1 tbs butter
- 2 c tomatoes, peeled and chopped
- ¾ c chopped bell pepper
- ¾ c chopped onion
- ¾ c chopped celery
- 1½ tsp minced garlic

Melt butter over medium heat and sauté the celery, bell pepper, and onion until the onions are translucent. Add the tomatoes and spices and simmer 20 to 30 min. Serves four.

This sauce is great for dressing up pre-cooked shrimp, fish, or chicken; or sauté your own meat, adding the sauce and simmering for a few minutes before serving. I even like to use a serving of this sauce over omelets for breakfast.

Calories per Serving	Calcium (mg)	Folate (mcg)	Zinc (mg)	Fiber (g)	Protein (g)	Predicted % Omega-6
86	39	36	0	3	2	67

Overall Fat (g)	Saturated Fat (g)	Cholesterol (mg)	Short Omega-6 (mg)	Short Omega-3 (mg)	Long Omega-6 (mg)	Long Omega-3 (mg)
4	2	8	367	75	0	0

By itself, the sauce produces a percent long omega-6 value of 67 percent, but add 4 ounces of shrimp or 3 oz of snapper (3 oz) and the percent long omega-6 drops to around 35 percent. If you substitute a half-cup of roasted white-meat chicken in place of the seafood, you still have only 252 calories per dish, but the percent long omega-6 goes up to 69 percent.

Cajun Spice Mix

    10 tbs paprika

    3 tbs onion powder

    3 tbs garlic powder

    3 tbs ground red pepper

    2 tbs white pepper

    2 tbs black pepper

    2 tbs thyme

    1½ tbs oregano

Mix all ingredients and put in a container for storage. I use this on seafood, chicken, and pork. This recipe will make 26 tablespoons of spice mix. Serving size for calculation is 1 tbs.

Calories per Serving	Calcium (mg)	Folate (mcg)	Zinc (mg)	Fiber (g)	Protein (g)	Predicted % Omega-6
20	21	6	0	1	1	71

Overall Fat (g)	Saturated Fat (g)	Cholesterol (mg)	Short Omega-6 (mg)	Short Omega-3 (mg)	Long Omega-6 (mg)	Long Omega-3 (mg)
1	0	0	259	41	0	0

Kumquat Cranberry Compote

  6 kumquats, seeded and chopped

  2 tbs cranberries

  1 tbs syrup

  1 tsp of butter

Melt butter over medium heat and sauté the fruits until they soften. Add syrup. Serve over fish or meats.

Calories per Serving	Calcium (mg)	Folate (mcg)	Zinc (mg)	Fiber (g)	Protein (g)	Predicted % Omega-6
144	53	19	0	9	1	48

Overall Fat (g)	Saturated Fat (g)	Cholesterol (mg)	Short Omega-6 (mg)	Short Omega-3 (mg)	Long Omega-6 (mg)	Long Omega-3 (mg)
4	3	11	126	73	0	0

Mango Salsa

2 mangos, peeled, seeded, and chopped

2 green onions, chopped

1 clove garlic, minced

1 jalapeno pepper, minced

1 tbs chopped fresh cilantro

1 tbs onion, chopped

1 chipotle pepper, minced

1 tbs fresh lime juice

salt and pepper to taste

Chop the mango into ½-inch cubes and combine with the remaining ingredients. Let sit for 1 hour. Drain any excess liquid and refrigerate until serving. Serves eight.

Calories per Serving	Calcium (mg)	Folate (mcg)	Zinc (mg)	Fiber (g)	Protein (g)	Predicted % Omega-6
41	10	12	0	1	1	36

Overall Fat (g)	Saturated Fat (g)	Cholesterol (mg)	Short Omega-6 (mg)	Short Omega-3 (mg)	Long Omega-6 (mg)	Long Omega-3 (mg)
0	0	0	19	20	0	0

Lemon Dill Butter

   1 stick (8 tbs) butter

   2 tbs chopped fresh dill

   1 tsp lemon zest

Soften butter and mix in chopped dill and lemon zest. Form butter into 1-inch balls. Wrap in plastic wrap and freeze. Use this butter on fish, chicken, or vegetables. Makes 10 tablespoons; serving size is 1 tbs.

Calories per Serving	Calcium (mg)	Folate (mcg)	Zinc (mg)	Fiber (g)	Protein (g)	Predicted % Omega-6
81	3	1	0	0	0	53

Overall Fat (g)	Saturated Fat (g)	Cholesterol (mg)	Short Omega-6 (mg)	Short Omega-3 (mg)	Long Omega-6 (mg)	Long Omega-3 (mg)
9	6	25	207	133	0	0

Sour Cream Cilantro Sauce

    1 c low-fat sour cream

    2 tbs lemon juice

    2 tbs finely chopped fresh cilantro

    1 tbs finely chopped onion

    1 tsp ground cumin

    ½ tsp hot sauce

Mix all ingredients in a bowl. Refrigerate until needed. Makes about 20 servings of one tablespoon. This sauce makes a good substitute for mayonnaise on sandwiches. It is also a great topping for black bean burgers.

Calories per Serving	Calcium (mg)	Folate (mcg)	Zinc (mg)	Fiber (g)	Protein (g)	Predicted % Omega-6
17	14	2	0	0	0	53

Overall Fat (g)	Saturated Fat (g)	Cholesterol (mg)	Short Omega-6 (mg)	Short Omega-3 (mg)	Long Omega-6 (mg)	Long Omega-3 (mg)
1	1	5	37	21	0	0

You can make the same sauce with plain fat-free Greek yogurt as well:

Calories per Serving	Calcium (mg)	Folate (mcg)	Zinc (mg)	Fiber (g)	Protein (g)	Predicted % Omega-6
8	26	2	0	0	1	54

Overall Fat (g)	Saturated Fat (g)	Cholesterol (mg)	Short Omega-6 (mg)	Short Omega-3 (mg)	Long Omega-6 (mg)	Long Omega-3 (mg)
0	0	0	5	0	0	0

Breads

Flax French Bread

   3 c all-purpose flour

   1 package of yeast

   ¼ c milled flax seed

   1 tsp salt

   1 c warm water

   1 egg white

Combine half of the flour in a bowl with the yeast, flax seed, and salt. Add water and stir in as much of the remaining flour as possible in a mixer with a dough attachment. Place dough ball on a lightly floured surface and knead for 8 to 10 minutes. Dough ball should be smooth and elastic. Place dough ball into a greased bowl in a warm place, cover, and let rise until it doubles in size. Punch down and roll out on a lightly floured surface. Cover and let rise for 10 to 15 minutes. Shape into a long, tapered loaf and place on a lightly greased and floured baking pan. Beat egg white with a tablespoon of water and brush loaf with egg white. Cover and let rise until it has doubled in size. Make 2 or 3 diagonal cuts in the top about a ¼-inch deep and bake at 375° for about 40 minutes, brushing again with egg white mixture after 15 to 20 minutes. Test bread for doneness, remove from oven, and cool on a wire rack.

Calories per Serving	Calcium (mg)	Folate (mcg)	Zinc (mg)	Fiber (g)	Protein (g)	Predicted % Omega-6
261	23	155	1	4	8	31

Overall Fat (g)	Saturated Fat (g)	Cholesterol (mg)	Short Omega-6 (mg)	Short Omega-3 (mg)	Long Omega-6 (mg)	Long Omega-3 (mg)
3	0	0	523	1,184	0	0

One-sixth of this loaf (about 4 inches) is 261 calories and 32 percent omega-6.

Kumquat Cranberry Bread

I developed this recipe to make use of all the kumquats we have growing in our back yard. It is a great breakfast bread and healthy as well.

2 c kumquats, seeded and chopped

3 eggs

1 c rolled oats

½ tsp salt

3 tbs coconut oil

1½ c flour, white enriched, self-rising

¼ c fat-free milk

1 c dried cranberries

1 tbs vanilla extract

1 tbs of ground cinnamon

1 c sucralose

1 c milled flax seed

¼ c agave nectar

2 tbs yeast

Mix all ingredients and pour into two 9-inch loaf pans that have been sprayed with nonstick cooking spray. Bake at 325° for about 30 minutes. The batter can also be baked as muffins.

Calories per Serving	Calcium (mg)	Folate (mcg)	Zinc (mg)	Fiber (g)	Protein (g)	Predicted % Omega-6
146	90	80	1	5	5	38

Overall Fat (g)	Saturated Fat (g)	Cholesterol (mg)	Short Omega-6 (mg)	Short Omega-3 (mg)	Long Omega-6 (mg)	Long Omega-3 (mg)
5	2	23	515	1,182	8	2

This recipe makes 2 loaves and, when cut into 12 slices per loaf, each slice is 146 calories.

Flax Tortilla

 1½-c flour, white enriched, self-rising

 ¼ c milled flax seed

 3 tbs butter, melted

 ½ c water

Mix together flour and flax seed, add melted butter, and mix with hands until flour is in small crumbs. Add water and mix. Place dough on a lightly floured surface and knead until dough is smooth and elastic. Divide into 8 small balls and roll out into thin round tortillas. Cook in a hot skillet until bubbly and lightly browned on both sides.

Calories per Serving	Calcium (mg)	Folate (mcg)	Zinc (mg)	Fiber (g)	Protein (g)	Predicted % Omega-6
147	14	59	0	2	3	31

Overall Fat (g)	Saturated Fat (g)	Cholesterol (mg)	Short Omega-6 (mg)	Short Omega-3 (mg)	Long Omega-6 (mg)	Long Omega-3 (mg)
6	3	12	398	946	0	0

These flour tortillas are great for burritos and sandwich or breakfast wraps and are significantly lower in omega-6 than most breads.

Tip: Roll out tortillas on a piece of wax paper or parchment paper; transfer the tortilla to the skillet to cook while still on the paper (tortilla side down). The paper will peel off easily after a few seconds; you can reuse the paper for the next tortilla. This tip eliminates the problem of the tortilla tearing while trying to lift and transfer it to the pan.

Yam Biscuits

    3 c flour, white enriched, self-rising

    2 c yams, cooked and mashed

    ¼ c milled flax seed

    ½ tsp cinnamon

    ¾ c fat-free milk

Mix all ingredients in a bowl until well mixed. Roll dough out to a 1-inch thickness, cut biscuits and place on a non-stick baking sheet. Bake at 425 for 10 to 12 minutes.

Calories per Serving	Calcium (mg)	Folate (mcg)	Zinc (mg)	Fiber (g)	Protein (g)	Predicted % Omega-6
110	96	52	0	2	3	30

Overall Fat (g)	Saturated Fat (g)	Cholesterol (mg)	Short Omega-6 (mg)	Short Omega-3 (mg)	Long Omega-6 (mg)	Long Omega-3 (mg)
1	0	0	211	517	0	0

A tablespoon of milled flax in this recipe makes 18 biscuits that are 100 calories each and just 42 percent omega-6. Adding ¼ c milled flax seed to the recipe drops the omega-6 drops to 30 percent. The flax seed adds only 10 calories per biscuit.

Flax Crackers

    1½ c white, enriched, self-rising flour

    ½ c milled flax seed

    3 tbs coconut oil

    ½ c water

    ½ tsp salt

    ¼ c Parmesan cheese

Mix flour, flax seed, and coconut oil until evenly mixed. Add water, mix ,and turn out onto a lightly flowered surface. Knead until smooth. Divide into 4 equal pieces and roll out into a sheet less than 1/8 inch thick. Transfer each sheet to a piece of aluminum foil, sprinkle with salt and Parmesan cheese. Score into approximately 1-inch squares. Bake at 250° for about 30 minutes. Break into crackers and allow to cool. If crackers are not crisp they may need to be returned to the oven for 15 to 20 minutes. Makes 8 servings.

Calories per Serving	Calcium (mg)	Folate (mcg)	Zinc (mg)	Fiber (g)	Protein (g)	Predicted % Omega-6
147	14	59	0	2	3	31

Overall Fat (g)	Saturated Fat (g)	Cholesterol (mg)	Short Omega-6 (mg)	Short Omega-3 (mg)	Long Omega-6 (mg)	Long Omega-3 (mg)
6	3	12	398	946	0	0

Desserts

Banana Pudding

　　1 package of instant pudding mix (sugar free, fat-free)

　　2 c milk (fat-free)

　　1 c chopped bananas

Make pudding according to package directions. Pour over chopped bananas. Refrigerate to let set. Serves four.

Calories per Serving	Calcium (mg)	Folate (mcg)	Zinc (mg)	Fiber (g)	Protein (g)	Predicted % Omega-6
102	154	13	1	1	5	34

Overall Fat (g)	Saturated Fat (g)	Cholesterol (mg)	Short Omega-6 (mg)	Short Omega-3 (mg)	Long Omega-6 (mg)	Long Omega-3 (mg)
0	0	0	27	15	0	0

This dish has just 102 calories per serving and 34 percent omega-6.

You can do the same thing with any other fruits. If you like, you can add chia seeds for added texture, protein, and fiber.

Chia Pudding

This pudding can be made with a wide variety of fruits or other flavors, like chocolate or vanilla. Chia seeds will soak up the liquid and make a gel that thickens in about 30 minutes. Chia seeds are high in protein and fiber, and the fat in chia seeds is about 55 percent omega-3.

 1 c strawberries (fresh or frozen)

 1/2 c chia seeds

 1 can of coconut milk

 1 tbs of agave nectar or a low-calorie sweetener like stevia.

Blend strawberries in coconut milk, stir in chia seeds, and let set for 30 minutes. Serves eight.

Calories per Serving	Calcium (mg)	Folate (mcg)	Zinc (mg)	Fiber (g)	Protein (g)	Predicted % Omega-6
118	116	23	1	1	4	45

Overall Fat (g)	Saturated Fat (g)	Cholesterol (mg)	Short Omega-6 (mg)	Short Omega-3 (mg)	Long Omega-6 (mg)	Long Omega-3 (mg)
5	2	4	509	585	0	0

This recipe has 167 calories and 46 percent omega-6 per serving. Milk can be used in place of the coconut milk. If skim milk is used, the calories are just 110 and the omega-6 is 44 percent. Whole milk produces 118 calories and 45 percent omega-6.

Strawberries and Whipped Cream

    1 c sliced strawberries

    1 tsp sugar-free sweetener, such as stevia

    2 tsp Grape Nuts cereal

    1 tsp milled flax seed

    1 piece of dark chocolate

    1 c whipped cream

For individual servings, place ½ cup of strawberries in a bowl and top with sweetener, Grape Nuts, and milled flax seed. Top each with a ½ cup of whipped cream and then shave a piece of dark chocolate over the whipped cream.

Calories per Serving	Calcium (mg)	Folate (mcg)	Zinc (mg)	Fiber (g)	Protein (g)	Predicted % Omega-6
139	45	28	0	3	2	51

Overall Fat (g)	Saturated Fat (g)	Cholesterol (mg)	Short Omega-6 (mg)	Short Omega-3 (mg)	Long Omega-6 (mg)	Long Omega-3 (mg)
8	5	23	249	162	0	0

This is one of our favorite desserts and we have it almost every night during the strawberry season. Each serving is just 159 calories and 34% omega-6.

Blueberries and Whipped Cream

  ½ c fresh blueberries

  1 tbs blueberry pie filling (see recipe below)

  2 tsp Grape Nuts cereal

  1 tsp milled flax seed

  1 piece of dark chocolate

  ½ c whipped cream

Combine the blueberries, pie filling, Grape Nuts, and flax seed. Top with ½ cup of whipped cream and shave a little dark chocolate on top.

Calories per Serving	Calcium (mg)	Folate (mcg)	Zinc (mg)	Fiber (g)	Protein (g)	Predicted % Omega-6
139	14	17	0	3	2	50

Overall Fat (g)	Saturated Fat (g)	Cholesterol (mg)	Short Omega-6 (mg)	Short Omega-3 (mg)	Long Omega-6 (mg)	Long Omega-3 (mg)
4	2	4	139	70	0	0

Blueberry Pie Filling

    1 c blueberries (fresh or frozen)

    ¼ c water

    2 tbs cornstarch

    1 c sugar

    1 tbs butter

    1 oz lemon juice

Mix water, cornstarch, and sugar in a saucepan. Add blueberries and cook over medium heat until sauce turns dark and thickens. Remove from heat, add butter and lemon juice, and stir until butter is melted. Makes a little over one cup, or 16 tablespoons. Calculations are based on a 1 tbs serving.

Calories per Serving	Calcium (mg)	Folate (mcg)	Zinc (mg)	Fiber (g)	Protein (g)	Predicted % Omega-6
32	1	1	0	0	0	42

Overall Fat (g)	Saturated Fat (g)	Cholesterol (mg)	Short Omega-6 (mg)	Short Omega-3 (mg)	Long Omega-6 (mg)	Long Omega-3 (mg)
0	0	1	18	11	0	0

Sautéed Bananas with Ice Cream

    1 medium banana

    1 c orange juice

    1 tsp ground cinnamon

    1 tsp vanilla extract

    Light vanilla ice cream

Peel and split banana. Pour orange juice into a non-stick frying pan, add banana, cinnamon, and vanilla extract, and cook until orange juice begins to thicken. Top each half of banana with a scoop of light vanilla ice cream and serve. Serves two.

Calories per Serving	Calcium (mg)	Folate (mcg)	Zinc (mg)	Fiber (g)	Protein (g)	Predicted % Omega-6
211	123	53	0	2	4	46

Overall Fat (g)	Saturated Fat (g)	Cholesterol (mg)	Short Omega-6 (mg)	Short Omega-3 (mg)	Long Omega-6 (mg)	Long Omega-3 (mg)
3	2	9	141	73	0	0

Snacks

Chocolate Chia Coconut Balls

¼ c chia seeds

2 tbs fig preserves or ¼ c dates

1 tbs cocoa powder

1 oz shredded coconut

Mash fig preserves with a fork. Add cocoa powder and chia seeds and mix into a thick paste. Roll into a log and slice into 6 pieces. Roll each piece into a ball and coat with shredded coconut.

Calories per Serving	Calcium (mg)	Folate (mcg)	Zinc (mg)	Fiber (g)	Protein (g)	Predicted % Omega-6
73	53	12	1	1	2	45

Overall Fat (g)	Saturated Fat (g)	Cholesterol (mg)	Short Omega-6 (mg)	Short Omega-3 (mg)	Long Omega-6 (mg)	Long Omega-3 (mg)
4	2	0	326	365	0	0

These chia balls can be made with a variety of flavors. You can add dried cranberries, dates, or any other dried fruit. You can also flavor them with cinnamon, vanilla, or other flavorings.

Fruit Chia Snacks

¼ c chia seeds

2 tbs strawberry preserves

5 dates

2 tbs cocoa powder

4 oz shredded coconut

Mash dates and mix with preserves, cocoa powder, and chia seeds. Sprinkle wax paper with about half of the coconut, then spread the date mixture over the shredded coconut as thinly as possible. Sprinkle the remaining coconut over the date mixture. Allow to set and dry. Refrigerate until serving.

Calories per Serving	Calcium (mg)	Folate (mcg)	Zinc (mg)	Fiber (g)	Protein (g)	Predicted % Omega-6
142	91	22	1	1	3	45

Overall Fat (g)	Saturated Fat (g)	Cholesterol (mg)	Short Omega-6 (mg)	Short Omega-3 (mg)	Long Omega-6 (mg)	Long Omega-3 (mg)
6	4	0	498	557	0	0

When divided into 8 pieces, these snacks are 142 calories each.

***

A Month of Menus

The menus that follow are typical of what I have eaten on this diet. The daily calorie intake ranges from about 1,200 calories to approximately 1,600 calories. I have a fairly light activity level and have been losing approximately 2 to 3 pounds per month on this diet. If you are not trying to lose weight or have a higher activity level, you can simply increase the serving size to obtain the calorie intake you need.

Week 1

Monday

Breakfast: Egg-white omelet w/Creole sauce, milk | 203 calories

Lunch: Imitation crab with sour cream cilantro sauce | 104 calories

Dinner: Red beans and rice, ham (3 oz) | 423 calories

Snacks: Blueberry yogurt (low-fat) | 225 calories

Dessert: Fruit salad with whipped cream | 176 calories

Daily Totals: 1,079 calories, 38 percent long omega-6

Tuesday

Breakfast: Blueberry oatmeal with flax seed | 193 calories

Lunch: Squash soup, tomato arugula salad |169 calories

Dinner: Seafood andouille gumbo | 472 calories

Snacks: Mango, banana, 2 oz cheddar cheese | 473 calories

Daily Totals: 1,306 calories, 33 percent long omega-6

Wednesday

Breakfast: Cottage cheese with strawberries, turkey sausage link, 8 oz orange juice | 259 calories

Lunch: Fish soup | 171 calories

Dinner: Squash casserole, 8 oz roasted chicken, 2 slices of Swiss cheese, green beans | 639 calories

Snacks: Watermelon wedge, peach | 134 calories

Daily Totals: 1,201 calories, 43 percent long omega-6

Thursday

Breakfast: Greek yogurt with blueberries | 195 calories

Lunch: Salad with tuna | 452 calories

Dinner: Ham steak, sweet potato, broccoli | 300 calories

Snacks: Honeydew melon, Gouda cheese, pineapple | 306 calories

Daily Totals: 1,253 calories, 40 percent omega-6

Friday

Breakfast: Flax pancakes, banana | 263 calories

Lunch: Spinach feta pizza | 292 calories

Dinner: Pasta with clams | 604 calories

Snacks: Mango, chia pudding | 304 calories

Daily Totals: 1,462 calories, 32% long omega-6

Saturday

Breakfast: Scrambled egg and cheese burrito | 297 calories

Lunch: Shrimp cocktail, tomato cucumber salad | 298 calories

Dinner: Chicken broccoli casserole | 447 calories

Snacks: ½ c vanilla ice cream (light), ½ c strawberries, 2 plums | 185 calories

Daily Totals: 1,232 calories, 34% long omega-6

Sunday

Breakfast: Uncle Sam cereal w/skim milk | 281 calories

Lunch: Black bean burger | 248 calories

Dinner: Braised pork loin (3 oz) with kumquat cranberry compote, Red cabbage with apples | 372 calories

Snacks: Apple, 1 c blueberries, 2 oz brie | 351 calories

Daily Totals: 1,523 calories, 34% long omega-6 (estimated—Uncle Sam cereal not listed)

Week 2

Monday

Breakfast: Egg-white omelet with cheese | 186 calories

Lunch: Salad with shrimp | 268 calories

Dinner: Burrito Supreme (with flax tortilla) | 542 calories

Snacks: Apple with cheese, mango | 405 calories

Dessert: Fruit salad with whipped cream | 176 calories

Daily Totals: 1,400 calories, 40% long omega-6

Tuesday

Breakfast: Kumquat cranberry bread, banana | 255 calories

Lunch: Chili with beans (and 1 tbs flax seed) | 308 calories

Dinner: Fish with mango salsa, rice, and broccoli | 401 calories

Snacks: Pretzel chips, Mandarin orange | 145 calories

Daily Totals: 1,139 calories and 35% long omega-6

Wednesday

Breakfast: Oatmeal with flax seed and blueberries | 193 calories

Lunch: Tossed salad, feta cheese, zero-calorie dressing | 254 calories

Dinner: Ham steak (3 oz), Skeet Taters, turnip greens | 344 calories

Snacks: Apple, 2 oz cheddar cheese | 310 calories

Dessert: Strawberries and whipped cream | 139 calories

Daily Totals: 1,240 calories, 58% long omega-6

Thursday

Breakfast: Grapefruit with Splenda, banana | 215 calories

Lunch: Flax tortilla w/chicken, spinach, feta | 406 calories

Dinner: Breaded duck breast with Creole sauce, pasta | 686 calories

Snacks: Banana, Gouda cheese (1 oz) | 210 calories

Daily Totals: 1,408 calories, 67% long omega-6

Friday

Breakfast: Egg-white omelet | 204 calories

Lunch: Pasta with clams & arugula in cream sauce | 212 calories

Dinner: Mushroom chicken, creamed cauliflower, spinach | 356 calories

Snacks: 2 oz pretzel chips, 2 oz Gouda cheese, apple | 499 calories

Dessert: Blueberries with whipped cream | 208 calories

Daily Totals: 1,559 calories, 45 % long omega-6

Saturday

Breakfast: Cottage cheese with fruit salad, yam biscuit | 359 calories

Lunch: Salad with chicken | 234 calories

Dinner: Vegetable chili, baked potato with cheese and sour cream | 628 calories

Snacks: Pear, 2 slices of canned pineapple | 154 calories

Dessert: Frozen yogurt | 115 calories

Daily Totals: 1,490 calories, 49% long omega-6

Sunday

Breakfast: Egg-white burrito with cheese | 297 calories

Lunch: Black bean burger w/ sour cream | 268 calories

Dinner: Mango salsa shrimp, broccoli, Skeet Taters | 505 calories

Snacks: Swiss cheese (2 oz) and fat-free crackers (6) | 329 calories

Dessert: Strawberries and whipped cream | 139 calories

Daily Totals: 1,539 calories, 27 % long omega-6

Week 3

Monday

Breakfast: Flax pancakes with fruit salad | 307 calories

Lunch: Arugula salad with tomatoes and feta | 97 calories

Dinner: Lentil soup with ham (3 oz), cabbage, Skeet Taters | 383 calories

Snacks: Chia ball, mango | 308 calories

Dessert: Strawberry ice cream (4 oz) | 127 calories

Daily Totals: 1,221 calories, 43% long omega-6

Tuesday

Breakfast: Scrambled egg with cheese, orange juice | 327 calories

Lunch: Tossed salad with sardines and balsamic vinegar | 257 calories

Dinner: Chili with beans | 308 calories

Snacks: Apple, Mandarin orange, chia ball | 192 calories

Dessert: Chia pudding | 169 calories

Daily Totals: 1,252 calories, 44% long omega-6

Wednesday

Breakfast: Uncle Sam cereal, skim milk, fruit salad | 434 calories

Lunch: Chicken burrito with flax tortilla | 437 calories

Dinner: Shrimp kabobs, rice, tomato cucumber onion salad | 352 calories

Snacks: Gouda cheese (1 oz), nectarine | 168 calories

Daily Totals: 1,656 calories, 37% long omega-6

Thursday

Breakfast: Orange juice, yam biscuit with butter & jelly | 313 calories

Lunch: Imitation crab salad with sour cream cilantro in a flax tortilla | 224 calories

Dinner: Chicken broccoli cheese casserole, butternut squash | 358 calories

Snacks: Mango, banana, cheddar cheese (2 oz) | 473 calories

Dessert: Blueberries and whipped cream | 208 calories

Daily Totals: 1,539 calories, 30% long omega-6

Friday

Breakfast: Greek yogurt and fruit salad | 280 calories

Lunch: Chicken, spinach, & feta tortilla pizza | 353 calories

Dinner: Creamy shrimp pasta | 601 calories

Snacks: Apple, Gouda cheese (2 oz) | 283 calories

Dessert: Chocolate ice cream | 143 calories

Daily Totals: 1,660 calories, 32% long omega-6

Saturday

Breakfast: Flax pancakes with butter, fruit salad | 307 calories

Lunch: Chicken burrito | 287 calories

Dinner: Stir-fried pork | 411 calories

Snacks: Pear, Swiss cheese (1 oz) | 336 calories

Dessert: Strawberries and whipped cream | 139 calories

Daily Totals: 1,545 calories, 44% long omega-6

Sunday

Breakfast: Fat-free cottage cheese and fruit salad | 249 calories

Lunch: Squash soup, yam biscuit with ham (3 oz) | 292 calories

Dinner: Roasted chicken (½ c), spinach, baked potato with butter and sour cream | 650 calories

Snacks: Pineapple, banana | 241 calories

Dessert: Chocolate pudding | 158 calories

Daily totals: 1,568 calories, 47% long omega-6

Week 4

Monday

Breakfast: Egg-white omelet with peppers, turkey sausage (2 links) | 315 calories

Lunch: Smoked fish spread on rye crackers (1 oz) | 312 calories

Dinner: Black bean burger on a bed of lettuce, with tomatoes and sour cream cilantro sauce | 383 calories

Snacks: Apple, Gouda cheese (2 oz) | 283 calories

Dessert: Sautéed bananas | 239 calories

Daily Totals: 1,504 calories, 41% long omega-6

Tuesday

Breakfast: Uncle Sam cereal w/skim milk, banana | 384 calories

Lunch: Oyster stew | 235 calories

Dinner: Shrimp Diane, tossed salad with feta | 107 calories

Snacks: Yogurt (low-fat w/fruit), plum, almonds (1 oz) | 341 calories

Dessert: Blackberries (½ c) and whipped cream | 94 calories

Daily Totals: 1,607 calories 37 % long omega-6

Wednesday

Breakfast: Blueberry oatmeal with flax seed | 193 calories

Lunch: Gumbo with rice | 472 calories

Dinner: Eggplant | 392 calories

Snacks: Apple, banana | 190 calories

Dessert: Strawberries and whipped cream | 139 calories

Daily Totals: 1,387 calories, 34 % long omega-6

Thursday

Breakfast: Egg-white omelet with cheese (1 oz) | 300 calories

Lunch: Flax French bread chicken sandwich (½)| 404 calories

Dinner: Stir-fried chicken with rice | 396 calories

Snacks: Gouda Cheese 2 oz, rye crackers (1 oz) | 306 calories

Dessert: Blueberries and whipped cream | 208 calories

Daily Totals: 1,599 calories, 49% long omega-6

Friday

Breakfast: Grapefruit w/Splenda, yam biscuit w/ham (2 oz) | 266 calories

Lunch: Spinach artichoke pasta with crab | 304 calories

Dinner: Jambalaya with shrimp and sausage | 601 calories

Snacks: Pretzels (2 oz), apple | 281 calories

Daily Totals: 1,482 calories, 33 % long omega-6

Saturday

Breakfast: Cottage cheese (1 c fat-free), ½ c mixed berries | 189 calories

Lunch: Arugula tomato feta salad, 4 oz roasted chicken | 218 calories

Dinner: Broiled Fish Parmesan, boiled red potatoes, broccoli | 529 calories

Snacks: Pear, banana | 231 calories

Dessert: Strawberries and whipped cream | 139 calories

Daily Totals: 1,274 calories, 31% long omega-6

Sunday

Breakfast: Greek yogurt (8 oz) with fruit salad | 290 calories

Lunch: Crab soup | 439 calories

Dinner: Chicken Florentine w/pasta, green beans | 680 calories

Snacks: Gouda cheese (1 oz), apple | 182 calories

Daily Totals: 1,723 calories, 38% long omega-6

Examples of Foods to Avoid

Traditional Breakfast

A traditional breakfast with 2 fried eggs, 3 strips of bacon, 2 slices of white toast, and a half-cup of white corn grits with a teaspoon of margarine clocks in at745 calories and 93% long omega-6.

Large Cheeseburger with Condiments and Veggies

1 large, single-patty cheeseburger contains 563 calories and produces 77 percent long omega-6. Adding a small bag of potato chips (2 oz) puts the calories at 867 and long omega-6 at 84%. Replace the potato chips with a large order of fries, and the calories jump to 1,141 with 78% omega-6.

Fried Chicken Sandwich

Even worse than a hamburger is a fried chicken sandwich, which generates 99% long omega-6. Adding a large order of fries adds 1,093 calories and generates 87% long omega-6.

Fried Fish Sandwich

A fried fish fillet on a plain hamburger bun with a tablespoon of mayonnaise and a leaf of lettuce weighs in at 424 calories and 75% long omega-6.

***

Lipids 101

These last sections are provided for those who want to understand the chemistry and biochemistry of lipids and eicosanoids, their production and metabolism, and their roles in our health. This section and the section on eicosanoids may be difficult to read for those not familiar with chemistry and biochemistry. You do not have to read and understand these sections, but as a scientist, this is the information that convinced me of the importance of this diet. While you may not be able to understand all of it, I do think it will help convince you of the importance of changing your oil.

Lipid chemistry is complex and extensive, so this short section will deal only with some of the most important forms and transformations related to eicosanoid production and its effects on our health. Lipids encompass a wide group of chemical classes, including cholesterols, triglycerides, phospholipids, sterols, fatty acids, and fat-soluble vitamins. They have a wide range of functions, including energy storage, energy production, and structural components of cells and signaling. They are the basic building blocks of a wide variety of hormones that affect many cellular functions. The production of eicosanoids is one of the most important functions of lipids in our bodies due to their involvement in inflammation, vasoconstriction, allergic response, and bronchioconstriction.

Fatty acids (FAs) are carboxylic acids with a long carbon tail that may be saturated (no double bonds) or unsaturated (containing double bonds in the long carbon tail). The unsaturated fatty acids are further divided into two groups: mono-unsaturated (containing only one double bond) and poly-unsaturated (containing two or more double bonds). All mammals use carbohydrates to synthesize FAs containing up to 16 carbon molecules through a process called lipogenesis. There are two 18-carbon fatty acids that are considered essential fatty acids (EFAs); this mean we must consume them from our diet because we cannot synthesize them. The two EFAs are alpha linolenic acid (ALA) and linoleic acid (LA). There are several others that are considered conditionally essential, like docosahexaenoic acid (DHA) and gamma linolenic acid (GLA).

There are two important forms of these FAs: omega-6 and omega-3 (Figure 1). The names omega-6 and omega-3 refer to the location of the double bonds. Omega-3 has the first double bond at the third carbon from the methyl end of the fatty acid (the end opposite the carboxylic acid group). Omega-6 has the first double bond at the sixth carbon from the methyl end. There are both mono-unsaturated and poly-unsaturated omega-3 and omega-6. However, only 18-carbon poly-unsaturated FAs can be converted to HUFAs. ALA is an omega-3, and LA is an omega-6 fatty acid.

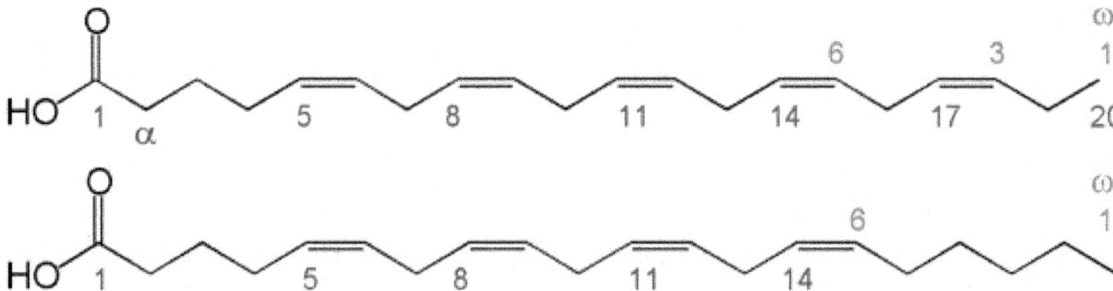

Figure 1. The chemical structures of eicosapentaenoic acid (EPA), an omega-3 HUFA with 5 double bonds starting at the third carbon from the methyl end, and arachidonic acid (AA), an omega-6 HUFA with 4 double bonds starting at the sixth carbon from the methyl end.

Figure 2 shows how mammals can convert the 18-carbon FAs into the more important acids: arachidonic acid (AA), a 20-carbon HUFA with 4 double bonds; eicosapentaenoic acid (EPA), a 20-carbon HUFA with 5 double bonds; docosahexaenoic acid (DHA), a 22- carbon HUFA with 6 double bonds; and di-homo-gamma-linoleic acid (DGLA), a 20-carbon HUFA with 3 double bonds. However, those conversions can be limited and affected by a variety of other factors, such as aging, insulin, and other lipids. We can also get these important HUFAs in our diet. The primary source of EPA and DHA is fish and shellfish, but they can also be found in marine algae and eggs. Arachidonic is found in all meats from mammals and poultry, but it can also be synthesized in our bodies from LA. DGLA can be synthesized in our bodies from GLA and LA. These four HUFAs (EPA, DHA, AA, and DGLA) are important precursors to the eicosanoids.

Eicosanoids are a group of lipid hormones produced from the 20- and 22-carbon HUFAs that are stored in our cells as part of the lipid bi-layer that forms the cell membranes.

Eicosanoids include prostaglandins, prostacyclins, leukotrienes, thromboxanes, and lipoxins. They are hormones—some call them super hormones—that regulate many basic physiological processes in our bodies, such as inflammation, blood pressure, clotting, immunity, and bronchioconstriction.

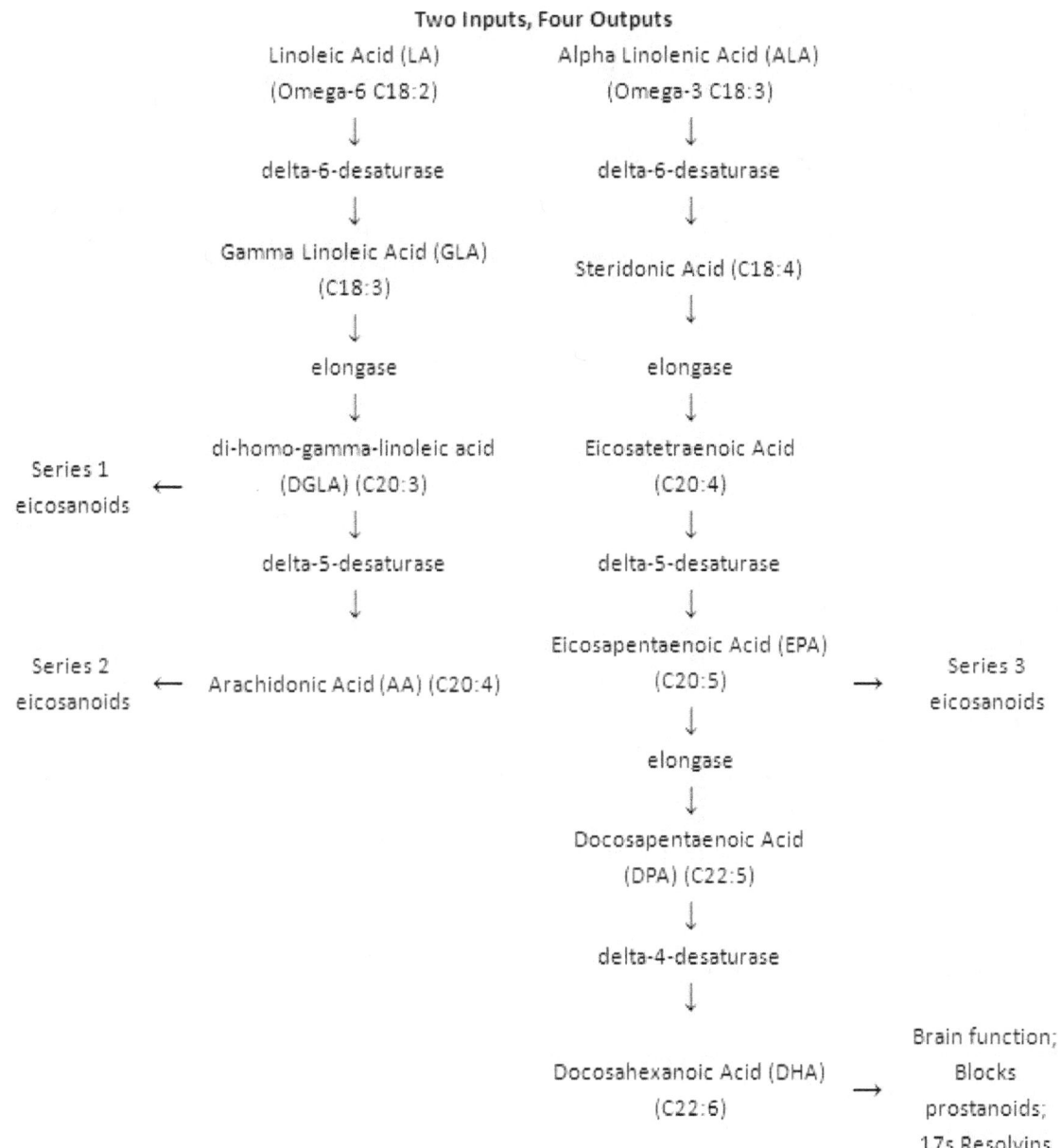

Two Inputs, Four Outputs

Linoleic Acid (LA)
(Omega-6 C18:2)
↓
delta-6-desaturase
↓
Gamma Linoleic Acid (GLA)
(C18:3)
↓
elongase
↓
di-homo-gamma-linoleic acid
(DGLA) (C20:3)
↓
delta-5-desaturase
↓

Series 1
eicosanoids ←

Series 2
eicosanoids ← Arachidonic Acid (AA) (C20:4)

Alpha Linolenic Acid (ALA)
(Omega-3 C18:3)
↓
delta-6-desaturase
↓
Steridonic Acid (C18:4)
↓
elongase
↓
Eicosatetraenoic Acid
(C20:4)
↓
delta-5-desaturase
↓
Eicosapentaenoic Acid (EPA)
(C20:5) → Series 3 eicosanoids
↓
elongase
↓
Docosapentaenoic Acid
(DPA) (C22:5)
↓
delta-4-desaturase
↓

Docosahexanoic Acid (DHA)
(C22:6) →

Brain function;
Blocks
prostanoids;
17s Resolvins

Figure 2. The metabolic pathways for conversion of linoleic acid (omega-6) and alpha linolenic acid (omega-3) to DGLA, AA, EPA and DHA—the four precursors to the eicosanoid hormones in our bodies.

***

Eicosanoids

Each of the different hormone groups, like prostaglandins or thromboxanes, are composed of several different compounds, the structure and biological effects of which varies depending on the location of the double bonds and oxygen-containing functional groups or linkages, but the most important distinction between these eicosanoids is whether it is derived from an omega-3 or an omega-6 HUFA. Those derived from omega-3 HUFAs (EPA and DHA) form the series 3 prostaglandins.

DGLA, an omega-6 HUFA, is used to form the series 1 prostaglandins. Both series 1 and series 3 prostaglandins are generally beneficial to our health. Series 2, which are derived from AA, another omega-6 HUFA, are generally detrimental. It is amazing how much difference the location of one double bond can make! The problem with DGLA is that it is a precursor to AA. Having a high level of insulin (which is common among Americans), increases the conversion rate of DGLA to AA.

The omega-6 eicosanoids formed from AA are associated with many of the common diseases and health problems we face in this country. We do need some of them for functions like clotting, fighting infection, and wound healing. This is good, since we can't totally avoid AA eicosanoids, but we need to keep the level low, at least below 50 percent. I have known for some time that prostaglandins are associated with inflammation, but what I learned from researching this diet is this is true only of prostaglandins derived from AA. Prostaglandins derived from EPA, DHA (series 3), or DGLA (series-1) are *anti*-inflammatory.

These different prostaglandins are given abbreviations like PGE1, PGE2, and PGE3; the number in these abbreviations refers to the series. In the first step of synthesis, PGHs are formed from EPA, DHA, or AA by the cyclooxygenase enzymes COX-1 and COX-2; other prostaglandins are then formed from the PGH. PGE1 inhibits platelet aggregation. PGE2, derived from AA, sensitizes pain neurons and increases pain as well as inducing fever. The COX enzymes are the targets of Non-Steroidal Anti-Inflammatory Drugs (NSAIDs) that are used to reduce inflammation by blocking the enzymes. The NSAIDs that we take inhibit both COX-1 and COX-2 enzymes, preventing the formation of both good and bad prostaglandins.

The hormones derived from the HUFAs are involved in many other processes in addition to inflammation, such as constriction or dilation of smooth muscle found in our arteries, aggregation or disaggregating of platelets, sensitivity of nerves, allergic response, depression, appetite, and regulation of other hormones. If we reduce the ratio of omega-6 to omega-3 HUFAs in our cells, we increase the ratio of good (anti-inflammatory) prostaglandins that are produced.

A number of the prostaglandins and their analogs are used pharmaceutically in medicine to treat problems such as glaucoma, asthma, and pulmonary hypertension, and to induce labor. PGE1 has strong vasodilating effects and is sold as the drug alprostadil for the treatment of erectile dysfunction and for the treatment of infants with circulatory problems.

Thromboxanes are derived from prostaglandin endoperoxides like PGH2 or PGH1. Thromboxanes are associated with the clotting and platelet aggregation processes that contribute to hardening of the arteries. Different thromboxanes are given abbreviations like TXA1, TXB1, TXA2, and TXA3; as with prostaglandins, the number refers to the series. Series 1 and 3 are derived from EPA, DHA, and DGLA and are beneficial. However, thromboxanes derived from AA increase aggregation and clotting, but they are important in preventing excessive bleeding and in the healing process. The only health problem I am aware of that is associated with low levels of omega-6 (levels around 30% omega-6), is excessive bleeding and an increase in the risk of strokes. Thromboxanes also affect heart rhythm—the series 2 thromboxanes can cause cardiac arrhythmia.

Leukotrienes are involved in the regulation of our immune system response. They are responsible for signaling neutrophils to adhere to endothelial cells and for stimulating secretion of lysosomal enzymes that cause much of the joint damage in arthritis. Leukotrienes can control smooth muscle contraction and are involved in both vasoconstriction and bronchioconstriction associated with asthma and allergies. Leukotrienes such as LTB4, derived from AA, have been implicated in chronic inflammation, such as arthritis. Leukotrienes such as LTB5, derived from EPA, limit the effects of LTB4. DGLA and its products can inhibit the production of leukotrienes from AA.

Lipoxins are derived from leukotrienes. All lipoxins, even those derived from AA, oppose the effects of leukotrienes, help resolve inflammation, and stimulate the synthesis of resolvins from omega-3 fatty acids. Essentially all of the eicosanoids derived from EPA, DHA, or DGLA are beneficial or have the effect of inhibiting or opposing the effects of eicosanoids derived from AA. The eicosanoids derived from AA are not inherently bad—many of their functions are important to good health. It is their excess that causes problems.

**

Glossary and Abbreviations

AA: Arachidonic acid, a 20-carbon omega-6 fatty acid or HUFA that is the precursor to series 2 eicosanoids. It is essential for life, but excessive amounts can cause or enhance many of our medical problems, such as high blood pressure, inflammation, arthritis, asthma, allergies, heart disease, and cardiac arrhythmia.

ALA: Alpha linolenic acid, a 18-carbon omega-3 fatty acid that can be used in our bodies to make EPA and DHA, the 20- and 22-carbon fatty acids that are precursors to beneficial series 3 eicosanoids. It is considered an essential fatty acid.

COX: Cyclooxygenase enzymes, COX-1 and COX-2, that are used to make prostaglandins from HUFAs in our bodies.

DGLA: Di-homo-gamma-linoleic acid, a 20-carbon omega-6 HUFA that is a precursor to the beneficial series 1 eicosanoids. It is made in our bodies from GLA and can be further metabolized into AA.

DHA: Docosahexaenoic acid, a 22-carbon omega-3 HUFA with 6 double bonds that is a precursor to beneficial eicosanoids and important to brain development in infants and brain health in adults.

Eicosanoids: This is the term that applies to a group of hormones or super hormones by individual cells. These hormones are used to signal other cells and promote various physiological responses, such as vasoconstriction, dilation, bronchioconstriction, allergy response, inflammation, nerve sensitivity, and clotting.

EPA: Eicosapentaenoic acid, a 20-carbon omega-3 fatty acid or HUFA with 5 double bonds. EPA is a precursor to the beneficial series 3 eicosanoids that are anti-inflammatory and help reduce blood pressure

FA: Fatty acids are carboxylic acids with a long carbon tail that may be saturated (no double bonds) or unsaturated (containing double bonds in the long carbon tail).

GLA: Gamma linoleic acid is a 18-carbon omega-6 fatty acid. It is a precursor to DGLA and can be made in our bodies from linoleic acid. It is also found in primrose oil, borage oil, and some safflower oils.

HDL: High Density Lipoprotein, the good form of cholesterol that helps prevent hardening of the arteries.

HUFA: Highly unsaturated fatty acid, this term applies to all of the eicosanoid precursors. The name is derived from the chemical term for 20, *eicos*.

KIM-2: The program that can calculate the percent long omega-6 HUFA that will result from the food that you eat. It is available to download at http://efaeducation.org/kim.html.

LA: Linoleic acid, an 18-carbon omega-6 fatty acid that can be used by our bodies to make DGLA and then AA. It is considered an essential fatty acid.

Lipids: These are various forms of fats in our bodies that include fatty acids, sterols, triglycerides, and eicosanoids.

NSAID: Non-steroidal anti-inflammatory drugs like aspirin and ibuprofen. These drugs inhibit the COX-1 and COX-2 enzymes used to make prostaglandins.

Omega-3: The term used to describe unsaturated fatty acids in which the first double bond starts at the third carbon from the methyl end of the fatty acid. The important omega-3 fats are ALA, EPA, and DHA. These are used to make beneficial eicosanoids.

Omega-6: The term used to describe unsaturated fatty acids in which the first double bond starts at the sixth carbon from the methyl end of the fatty acid. The important omega-6 fats are LA, DGLA, and AA.

PUFA: Poly-unsaturated fatty acids. These are fatty acids with 2 or more double bonds. Most vegetable oils are made of various PUFAs. Those that are 16-carbon or less cannot be used to make HUFAs or eicosanoids. The 18-carbon PUFAs are LA and ALA; they can be used in our bodies to make the 20- and 22-carbon HUFAs that our bodies use to make eicosanoids.

Prostaglandins: An important series of eicosanoid hormones that are involved in inflammatory response, fever, contraction and relaxation of smooth muscle, redness, and swelling. All prostaglandins contain 20 carbon atoms and a 5-carbon ring. They are often abbreviated, e.g., PGE1 for a prostaglandin with an epoxide ring belonging to the series 1 eicosanoids. Series-1 and series-3 prostaglandins are anti-inflammatory; series-2 prostaglandins are inflammatory.

Thromboxanes: A series of eicosanoid hormones involved in clotting and adhesion of blood cells. Thromboxanes are made from prostaglandins and are given abbreviations like TXA1. Series-1 and series-3 thromboxanes reduce platelet aggregation; series-2 thromboxanes increase aggregation or clotting.

Leukotrienes: A series of eicosanoid hormones associated with allergic responses. Those derived from AA, such as LTB4, increase allergic response. Those derived from EPA and DGLA inhibit the formation of LTB4.

Lipoxins: These are eicosanoids that are involved with anti-inflammatory and immuno-modulating response. Lipoxins are involved in the resolution of inflammation.

LDL: Low Density Lipoprotein, the bad cholesterol that causes hardening of the arteries

PLA: Phospholipase is the enzyme that clips 20-carbon HUFA lipids from the phospholipids that form a cell's lipid bilayer.

Recipe Abbreviations

c: cup

tsp: teaspoon

tbs: tablespoon

oz: ounce

lb: pound

pt: pint

***

Acknowledgements

I want to thank my wife and son for encouraging me to write this book. I also would like to thank Frank Abbott (frankabbott.com) for allowing me to use his photograph "Sunrise Over Emanuel Point" for my book cover. I thank Dr. Bill Lands for helping me to find information and his research that has changed my life. Thanks to all my friends and family for reviewing early versions and all their suggestions. And, last but not least, I would like to recognize Lee Ann Pingel (http://leeannpingel.writersresidence.com/) for editing this book.

http://efaeducation.org/kim.html

https://en.wikipedia.org/wiki/Eicosanoid

***

Notes

<u>1</u>. The KIM-2 program has a formula that estimates the percent that is converted to long omega-6 HUFAs. There is not a fixed percentage conversion rate for the C-18 FA to C-20 & 22 HUFAs; it is dependent on a variety of factors. The KIM-2 program uses 8 parameters to estimate the percent of long omega-6 that will be produced.

<u>2</u>. Lands, W.E. (2003). Diets Could Prevent Many Diseases. *Lipids* 38(4), 317−321.

<u>3</u>. The mathematical formula for the line in that graph is: CHD = 3 X (% omega-6) − 75 with a correlation coefficient of 0.99 (r2 = 0.98).

<u>4</u>. Lands, W.E., et al. (1992) Maintenance of lower proportions of (n - 6) eicosanoid precursors in phospholipids of human plasma in response to added dietary (n - 3) fatty acids. *Biochim. Biophys. Acta*, 1180(2):147−162.

<u>5</u>. Lands, W.E., and Lamoreaux, E. (2012) Using 3-6 differences in essential fatty acids rather than 3/6 ratios gives useful food balance scores. *Nutr Metab (Lond)* 9(1):46.

<u>6</u>. I am indebted to Dr. W.E. Lands for directing me to this website: http://www.drsears.com/ArticlePreview/tabid/399/itemid/66/Default.aspx

***

For Additional Information

http://www.drsears.com/ArticlePreview/tabid/399/itemid/66/Default.aspx

http://www.cs.stedwards.edu/chem/Chemistry/CHEM43/CHEM43/Eicosanoids/FUNCTION.HTML

http://www.jlr.org/content/46/5/949.full

http://www.tunedbody.com/heart-surgeon-declares-really-causes-heart-illness/#

http://omega-6-omega-3-balance.omegaoptimize.com/files/8/9/8/7/3/147167-137898/Lands_Omega_6_Handout.pdf

http://nutritiondata.self.com/facts/finfish-and-shellfish-products/4108/2

***

www.ingramcontent.com/pod-product-compliance
Lightning Source LLC
Chambersburg PA
CBHW080414290526

45791CB00008BA/2274